# THE LITTLE BOOK OF MUDRA MEDITATIONS

D1452581

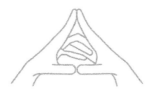

# THE
# LITTLE BOOK OF
# MUDRA
# MEDITATIONS

## 30 YOGA HAND GESTURES
## FOR HEALING

AUTUMN ADAMS

ROCKRIDGE
PRESS

For general information on our other products and services or to obtain technical support, please contact our Customer Care Department within the United States at (866) 744-2665, or outside the United States at (510) 253-0500.

Rockridge Press publishes its books in a variety of electronic and print formats. Some content that appears in print may not be available in electronic books, and vice versa.

Interior and Cover Designer: Diana Haas
Art Producer: Samantha Ulban
Editor: John Makowski
Production Editor: Jenna Dutton

Illustrations © Pelin Kahraman. Helen Stiriadis/Stocksy, cover. All other illustrations used under license © Shutterstock. Author photo courtesy © Alejandro Torres

ISBN: Print 978-1-64611-490-0 | eBook 978-1-64611-491-7
R0

This book is dedicated to my mom, who taught me that anything is possible, to my hubby for his continued support, and to my teachers, past, present, and future.

# Contents

# Introduction

Welcome to *The Little Book of Mudra Meditations*. I began my yoga journey as a high school student nearly 20 years ago. I am now a 500-hour certified yoga instructor, retreat leader, and yoga teacher trainer. I've been practicing mudras for as long as I have been teaching yoga.

I still remember my first "aha" moment with mudras. It was during a challenging, stressful period of my life. I was experiencing a ton of anxiety, wasn't sleeping well, and couldn't relax, or even close my eyes in *savasana* at the end of a yoga class. One evening at yoga class, the teacher taught us Ksepana Mudra (page 101), a mudra that helps us let go and surrender. I had such a strong, emotional, healing response to this mudra that I knew there was more to this practice. The breathwork, the mudra, and the meditation together gave me the insight and clarity I needed to realize I didn't have to control everything. Of course, my rational mind already knew this, but practicing the mudra helped me access the wisdom of my soul. The simple practice took me to a place of calm and centeredness.

Mudras are one of yoga's little hidden gems. They have the power to help us practice radical self-love, transform our relationships, and heal ourselves in a beautiful, simple, and holistic way. I've witnessed my students, by way of mudras, drop into the tenderness of their hearts, step into their personal power, and access their inner truths.

My hope is that this book will empower you to take your healing into your own hands. I hope that, within its pages, you will find the tools to unlock improved physical health, spiritual growth, and a joyful heart.

## How to Use This Book

The first part of this book lays the groundwork for the mudras and meditation practices included in the following chapters. You'll find an introduction to the five elements of Ayurveda, simple breathing exercises, and an exploration of each chakra. You'll discover what mudras and meditation are, how they work, and how they can help you on your path toward balance and healing.

The second portion of this book explains 30 of the most effective mudras for physical, emotional, and spiritual health. For each mudra, you will learn how to perform it, its purpose, which chakra(s) it affects, and any other benefits it provides. Under each mudra, you will find additional details on its origin, mythology, and modern application. Each mudra is followed by a guided meditation. Each meditation is specifically chosen to enhance the mudra it is paired with to provide the greatest possible benefit.

I encourage you to make these mudras and meditations your own. Try them as they are taught first, then explore their applications and make adaptations. Choose a mudra that resonates with you and work with it for an amount of time that feels right. Most importantly, remember these mudras are meant to be beacons of life, joy, and positivity, so be patient and kind with yourself as you embark on learning about this ancient tradition.

Whether this is the first time you've heard of mudras and meditation or you've been practicing yoga for years, the practices in this book are accessible to all. The great thing about mudras is that most of them can be done easily, at any time—during your morning commute, while walking the dog, on lunch break, in yoga class, or in meditation. There is no better time to start practicing than right now. No matter who you are or what you're dealing with, this book can help you on your way to balance, self-care, and healing.

CHAPTER ONE

# All About Mudras

W hat are mudras? Where do they come from? How can they
balance your chakras (energy centers in the body associated
with different physical and psychological characteristics),
enhance your meditation, and help you pursue healing, self-care, and
balance? When can you practice mudras? This chapter will explain
everything you need to know about these ancient yoga hand gestures and
how they can improve your well-being.

## What Are Mudras?

Mudras are yoga for your hands. In our yoga practice we use yoga poses,
called *asanas*, to improve our well-being. Much like asanas, we can use
hand mudras, or gestures, to help clear our mind, improve our health, find
ease in meditation, and cultivate peace and tranquility in our daily life.

Even if you've never done yoga before, you've likely seen some of the most common yoga mudras practiced. What the yogis call Anjali Mudra you would recognize as "prayer hands," and Jnana Mudra (page 67) is commonly depicted in images of Hindu deities and Western meditators.

## A BRIEF HISTORY OF MUDRAS

*Mudra* means "seal," "mark," or "gesture" in Sanskrit. If we look at the Sanskrit roots we see "mud," which translates as "joy," "happiness," or "delight," and "dru," which translates as "giving" or "bringing forth." Simply put, mudras are gestures that bring happiness, joy, and delight.

In this book we will focus on *hasta* mudras, or mudras of the hands. These mudras originated in ancient India and have been used for centuries in meditation, ritual, and classical dance. Although these hand mudras have their roots in Hinduism, Buddhism, and Jainism, symbolic gestures of the hands have been used by many different cultures. Religious and cultural icons throughout history have been depicted using gestures similar to the yoga mudras you will learn in this book.

Ayurveda, a science of self-healing, is often considered yoga's sister science. This 5,000-year-old holistic healing system addresses mental, physical, emotional, and spiritual well-being. Ayurveda recognizes five elements, and each element is associated with a different finger:

thumb = fire

index finger = air

middle finger = ether (differs from air, which is associated with our sense of touch and represents our capacity for motion, in that it is the essence of emptiness and is the most subtle of the elements)

ring finger = earth

pinky finger = water

These elements are groups of qualities and characteristics related to our physical being and our psychological makeup, different functions and actions, and even different tastes. For example, in the physical body, the different elements are associated with different tissues, organs, and specific functions of the body.

Consider the element fire, which is linked to digestion, energy creation, heat building, and action. In personality, it is our capacity to take action and the intensity of our actions.

Too much fire in the body = excessive sweating, rashes, inflammation, loose stools, and quickness to anger

Too little fire in the body = cold, sluggish digestion, and pale skin

When fire is "just right" and, therefore, balanced = bright eyes, radiant skin, digestion humming along nicely, and a sharp mind

Mudras are one way to bring these elements into balance for total health and well-being.

## THE BENEFITS OF MUDRAS

Mudras are an alternative way to bring vitality, ease, and tranquility into your life, to bring health to the whole person—both body and mind. By combining mudras with asanas, pranayama breathing exercises, and meditation, you are able to balance your chakras, clear blockages in energy flow, and direct that energy to create positive transformation so you can experience vibrant health and happiness.

When your energy is balanced, you reap numerous benefits, such as improved mental focus, emotional healing, better sleep, pain relief, increased energy, uplifted mood, stress release, and spiritual well-being. Practicing mudras helps you deepen self-love and improve your relationship with yourself and others. You become more joyous, compassionate, and loving. You vibrate at a higher level.

You can amplify the benefits of mudras by combining them with visualizations, pranayama, and meditation. Visualizations help create new, healthy patterns of thought and behavior. Pranayama increases your lung capacity and *prana*, or life-force energy. Meditation creates mental and emotional steadiness.

Mudras give you another tool to use on your path toward emotional and physical well-being and spiritual evolution. When you use mudras, you embody the specific qualities and energies associated with the mudra and its related elements and chakras. You unite the body, mind, and spirit, and they work together for your well-being.

Even if you pay no attention to yoga, chakras, or energy healing, mudras are still a great way to help you concentrate, focus on your breathing, and improve your meditation. Mudras are a simple practice you can use throughout the day, whether at home or in the office.

## Mudras and Chakras

*Chakra*, in Sanskrit, means "wheel"; therefore, chakras are wheels of energy where energy channels intersect. These energy channels carry our prana, or life-force energy, throughout our body and into the chakras. There are seven major chakras, or energy centers, located along the entire length of your spine. Each chakra corresponds to certain physical, emotional, and spiritual attributes. These chakras influence our perception of the world around us, and our behavior.

When our chakras are balanced, energy, or prana, flows freely within our body via energy channels known as *nadis*. If the chakras are unbalanced or blocked, energy may become trapped or restricted, and our entire being experiences disharmony and dis-ease—from the way we interact with others to our overall health.

Each of our fingers is associated with a different chakra (in addition to the elements we learned about on page 3); therefore, we're able to use specific mudras to redirect and guide the flow of prana (energy) to unblock, balance, and activate our chakras.

## THE ROOT CHAKRA

**Sanskrit name:** Muladhara

**Location:** Base of the spine

**Color:** Red

**Associated finger:** Ring finger

**Physical elements controlled:** Earth

**Emotional/spiritual elements controlled:** The root chakra governs our sense of safety, security, and stability; physical health; and our connection to our roots.

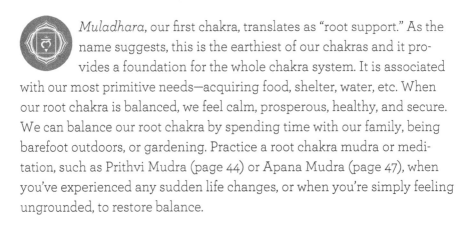

*Muladhara*, our first chakra, translates as "root support." As the name suggests, this is the earthiest of our chakras and it provides a foundation for the whole chakra system. It is associated with our most primitive needs—acquiring food, shelter, water, etc. When our root chakra is balanced, we feel calm, prosperous, healthy, and secure. We can balance our root chakra by spending time with our family, being barefoot outdoors, or gardening. Practice a root chakra mudra or meditation, such as Prithvi Mudra (page 44) or Apana Mudra (page 47), when you've experienced any sudden life changes, or when you're simply feeling ungrounded, to restore balance.

## THE SACRAL CHAKRA

**Sanskrit name:** Svadhisthana

**Location:** Sacrum

**Color:** Orange

**Associated finger:** Pinky finger

**Physical elements controlled:** Water

**Emotional/spiritual elements controlled:** The sacral chakra governs our ability to "go with the flow," adapt, and let go. It is associated with our creativity, pleasure, sexuality, and connection with others.

 Our second chakra, Svadhisthana, finds its roots in two Sanskrit words: "sva," or self, and "adhisthana," or abode. *Svadhisthana* is often translated as "one's own abode." As this chakra is closely related to our sexuality, it also governs our sexual organs and reproductive health. When the sacral chakra is balanced, we exude vitality, we have a healthy relationship with sensuality, and we are optimistic, uninhibited, and creative. If you find yourself feeling "stuck," or devoid of vitality, a sacral chakra mudra, such as Shakti Mudra (page 50) or Varuna Mudra (page 53), will help you feel like yourself again.

**Sanskrit name:** Manipura

**Location:** Navel and solar plexus

**Color:** Yellow

**Associated finger:** Thumb

**Physical elements controlled:** Fire

**Emotional/spiritual elements controlled:** The solar plexus chakra is associated with our inner strength, staying power, determination, fortitude, confidence, self-esteem, courage, integrity, and authority.

In Sanskrit, *Manipura* translates as the "dwelling place of gems." It is here that the gems of self-worth, integrity, leadership, courage, and fortitude reside. Along with ruling our personal power, the third chakra is associated with the digestion and assimilation of food and ideas. Manipura chakra is also the home of our ego. As Manipura chakra awakens and prana moves up through the chakras, we gradually transcend the ego. When our third chakra is balanced, we are radiant, dependable, respectful, and true to ourselves. If you're experiencing a lack of motivation or commitment, try practicing Pran Mudra (page 61).

**Sanskrit name:** Anahata

**Location:** Heart center

**Color:** Green

**Associated finger:** Index finger

**Physical elements controlled:** Air

**Emotional/spiritual elements controlled:** Our heart chakra is associated with love in all of its forms: self-love, compassion, forgiveness, gratitude, joy, acceptance, faith, and devotion.

 Anahata, our fourth chakra, is the chakra of the heart and the seat of Divine love. In Sanskrit, *Anahata* means "unstruck" or "unbeaten." As the middle chakra, Anahata is the bridge between the lower, earthier chakras and the upper, more ethereal chakras. When the fourth chakra is balanced, the gifts of Anahata are plentiful; these gifts include compassion, contentment, emotional balance, empathy, love, a sense of unity, and trust. Practice the Anahata Chakra Mudra (page 104) to heal a broken heart, work through fear, or to practice giving and receiving unconditional love.

**Sanskrit name:** Vishuddha

**Location:** Throat

**Color:** Turquoise

**Associated finger:** Middle

**Physical elements controlled:** Ether

**Emotional/spiritual elements controlled:** Our throat chakra is associated with communication, self-expression, creativity, deep listening, and our ability to speak our truth.

 In Sanskrit, *Vishuddha* means "especially pure." This chakra brings balance and harmony to opposites and moves us from an experience of duality to nonduality. When Vishuddha is balanced, your words and actions become aligned, you have a strong sense of self-knowledge, and you freely express yourself. When your throat chakra is underactive, you may find it difficult to express yourself for fear of judgment or failure, whereas if your fifth chakra is overactive, you may tend to speak over others, or struggle to listen. Practice a Vishuddha chakra mudra, such as Shunya Mudra (page 37) or Udana Vayu Mudra (page 111), for pure and honest communication and creative self-expression.

## THE THIRD-EYE CHAKRA

**Sanskrit name:** Ajna

**Location:** Midbrain, behind the center of the forehead

**Color:** Indigo

**Associated finger:** Palm

**Physical elements controlled:** Light

**Emotional/spiritual elements controlled:** Our third-eye chakra is related to intuition, insight, intellect, and clarity, in addition to our ability to dream and imagine.

In Sanskrit, *Ajna* translates as our center of "command." The sixth chakra is sometimes referred to by mystics as the seat of the soul because it connects us to a higher perspective, where we are able to see the big picture, interpret our dreams, create a personal vision, and receive knowledge from a higher source—whether spirit, God, Universal Wisdom, or something different. Mudras for the sixth chakra, such as Garuda Mudra (page 80) and Dhyana Mudra (page 74), can help you access a higher state of awareness and the knowledge, guidance, and direction of your inner guru.

## THE CROWN CHAKRA

**Sanskrit name:** Sahasrara

**Location:** Just above the crown of the head

**Color:** Violet

**Associated finger:** None

**Physical elements controlled:** Ether

**Emotional/spiritual elements controlled:** Our crown chakra is all about connecting with the Divine, which develops into spiritual unity, peace, bliss, understanding, and liberation.

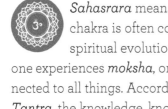 *Sahasrara* means "thousand-petaled" in Sanskrit. The highest chakra is often considered the seat of God/spirit/source. When spiritual evolution reaches Sahasrara at the crown of the head, one experiences *moksha*, or liberation from ignorance, and feels connected to all things. According to the ancient teachings of the *Kundalini Tantra*, the knowledge, knower, and known all become one. A balanced seventh chakra manifests as wisdom, open-mindedness, and the ability to integrate new information. If you're "stuck in your head" or disconnected from spirit or source, try incorporating a Sahasrara chakra mudra, such as Hakini Mudra (page 64) or Bija Mudra (page 70), into your daily routine.

## MUDRAS AS A COMPLEMENT TO CONVENTIONAL MEDICINE

Mudras are meant as a complement to conventional medicine, *not* as a replacement. You should *always* consult your doctors or other health care providers and receive their guidance regarding any health issue or special condition, including pregnancy, before beginning a new practice or exercise.

Although Western medicine offers valuable healing techniques such as antibiotics and surgery, it usually doesn't address health matters such as reducing stress or dealing with chronic pain—let alone spiritual or emotional health. That's where practices like yoga, meditation, and mudras come in. They work *with* conventional medicine, not *instead of* it.

If you experience pain or discomfort while practicing mudras, take a moment to pause and stretch. When you return to the mudra, know that it doesn't have to be perfect for you to receive its benefits.

### Remember to Breathe

How often are you fully aware of your breath? If you're like most people, you go through the majority of your day without much awareness of your breath at all. We're all constantly breathing, but most of us are doing it "wrong." How so? Without training and conscious effort, we tend to isolate our breath in our chest, we slouch forward at our computers, and are taught to suck in our belly—add a bit of stress to this way of breathing and we have a recipe for a breathing disaster. We become tense and tight and there is nowhere for the breath to go.

According to Dr. Jonathan P. Parsons, interim director of the Division of Pulmonary, Critical Care, and Sleep Medicine at the Ohio State University Wexner Medical Center, "In healthy people without chronic lung disease, even at maximum exercise intensity, we only use 70 percent of the possible lung capacity." If we're breathing significantly below our lung capacity, our heart has to work harder to pump oxygenated blood throughout the body.

Breathing happens automatically via our autonomic nervous system, but we are also able to control our breath via our voluntary nervous system. A recent review of 68 scientific studies analyzing the effects of pranayama published in the *Journal of Ayurveda and Integrative Medicine* found that pranayama can manipulate the parasympathetic nervous system (rest and digest response), the sympathetic nervous system (fight or flight response), blood pressure, and brain wave activity. Breathing correctly and efficiently improves our physical and mental health, providing us with less stress, improved energy, easier digestion, and better sleep.

Breathwork, in particular the pranayama techniques of yoga, are directly linked to the flow of prana in the body. Mudras and pranayama work hand in hand to amplify the benefits on our journey of self-care, healing, and balance.

## BREATHING DEEPLY: THREE-PART BREATH

In this section, you will learn how to maximize your lung capacity, gain control of your breath, and create a sense of tranquility.

1. Start by finding a comfortable seat. You can prop yourself up on a cushion or sit on the edge of a chair with your feet firmly planted on the ground and your ribs right above your pelvis. Sitting this way gives you access to your full breath capacity.
2. Bring your hands to your belly. With each inhale, breathe down to your belly and feel your belly expand into your hands. On each exhale breath, feel your belly soften.
3. Now bring your hands to the sides of your rib cage. Inhale and feel your belly expand and then your rib cage expand. Exhale and feel your rib cage and belly draw in.
4. Bring your hands to your collarbones. Breathe in and fill your lungs from the very bottom to the very top. Did you notice your collarbones lift? Exhale and empty your lungs from top to bottom.
5. Fill your lungs from bottom to top as you inhale; as you exhale, empty your lungs from top to bottom. Practice for 7 to 10 minutes.

## SQUARE BREATH

Square breath adds another layer of depth to your three-part breath (page 15). Square breathing has many of the same benefits as three-part breathing, including calming the nervous system, relieving tension and stress, and strengthening the immune system.

1. Find a comfortable seated position and bring your awareness to your breath. Begin to slow your breath. When square breathing, you might find it helpful to envision a square. Each portion of the breath makes up one side of the square.
2. Inhale for a count of four. Retain the breath for a count of four. Exhale for a count of four. Hold the breath for a count of four.

Inhale: 4, 3, 2, 1
Hold: 4, 3, 2, 1
Exhale: 4, 3, 2, 1
Hold: 4, 3, 2, 1

3. Complete a minimum of 10 rounds of square breath.

Make this practice your own by lengthening or shortening the sides of your "square." If you find you are gasping for breath, opt out of or shorten the breath retention until you feel more comfortable. *Breath retention practices are not advised for expectant mothers and those with glaucoma or uncontrolled high blood pressure.*

What is pranayama? "Prana" is energy; it is life force—and the breath is its vehicle. "Yama" is control. Pranayama teaches us fully conscious, controlled breathing. In hatha yoga, pranayama and mudras are practiced to awaken the dormant energy of Kundalini Shakti and send it upward through the chakras, awakening them as it flows up toward the crown.

## Meditating with Mudras

Mudras can be practiced at any time, including while watching television or sitting on the bus, but you'll reap the most rewards combining mudras with meditation. I've been known to practice mudras before having difficult discussions with loved ones or sitting in a business meeting. Some mudras we do naturally in these situations, for example placing your hands over your heart to show you care, or bringing your fingertips together when you're thinking intensely. But when I bring mudras into my meditation practice, I get the most benefits. It's when energy, attention, and intention align.

### THE BENEFITS OF MEDITATION

Meditation is the practice of training the mind. Through meditation we gain awareness, perspective, and clarity. We learn to practice nonattachment to our thoughts and the things we cannot control. The time we spend in meditation offers us a moment of introspection and an opportunity to be present with our thoughts without judgment. Thich Nhat Hanh, a Buddhist teacher, explains meditation as "offering your genuine presence to yourself in every moment."

Did you know that meditation is the fastest-growing health trend in the United States? According to a study by the Centers for Disease Control and Prevention (CDC), the number of meditation practitioners increased threefold between 2012 and 2017. This growing practice has its roots in Hinduism and Taoism and is a central tenet of Buddhism.

Meditation has numerous benefits, ranging from stress relief to increased focus, so it's no surprise the number of meditators in the United States has increased. And although relaxation may not be the goal of meditation, it is definitely one of its greatest benefits. Many meditation practitioners also experience improved sleep, increased happiness and contentment, and lowered sympathetic nervous system stimulation.

A 2011 study led by a team of Harvard-affiliated researchers at Massachusetts General Hospital reported that mindfulness meditation manifests changes in our brain that improve our well-being. For example, the study found that meditation increases gray matter density in the hippocampus, a region of the brain associated with learning, memory, self-awareness, compassion, introspection, and a decrease in brain matter in the amygdala, a portion of the brain associated with stress and anxiety. We can, literally, change our brain with meditation.

## MUDRAS AND MEDITATION

Each hand mudra offers a symbolic meaning that comes from a place of love and positivity. These simple gestures of the hands are an outward expression rooted in our inner intentions. Mudras are a means of communication between our body, mind, and spirit. By combining mudras and meditation we're able to magnify our positive intentions by releasing distracting thoughts and turning our awareness from the external to the internal. Meditation and mudras, when practiced together, combine our positive intention with inner awareness and mindfulness, resulting in calm, clarity, and personal transformation.

When you're beginning a meditation practice, it is helpful to have an object to focus your awareness on. Having an object to focus awareness on helps tame the "monkey mind," gives the mind something to do, and trains it for clarity and focus. Without the distractions of our mind, we're able to drop into the intelligence and wisdom of our heart. This "object" could be a mudra, an intention, an image, a mantra such as "om," or even your breath.

Mudras can enhance our meditation practice by providing a single point of focus for the mind. With practice, this one-pointed focus in meditation helps improve our focus, concentration, and mind-set when we're facing "real-world" tasks such as job deadlines, homework assignments, and even household chores. For example, if I have a big deadline coming up, and my mind is spinning and I'm completely stressed out, I take a few minutes to drop into a meditation with Ksepana Mudra (page 101) and know that I can shift my mind-set into a more positive space, reduce my stress levels, and refocus.

On the other hand, meditation creates space for healing by freeing our mind of distractions and, again, quieting the "monkey mind" that normally jumps from idea to idea and thought to thought. It's in this space of quiet and stillness that the benefits of a mudra practice really shine. When the mind is calm and clear, we have the capacity to heal. By closing the energetic circuits of prana, or energy, at the fingertips, we're able to guide the subtle energies of the mudras and the flow of prana back into the body and bring balance to the elements and chakras.

# HEALTHY HANDS: MASSAGE

Throughout this book you will find sidebars with stretches and exercises to keep your hands, wrists, and shoulders happy and healthy. Here is an awesome hand massage to get you started.

Bring the palms of your hands together and briskly rub them together until they become warm. When your hands are nice and toasty, rub your warm hands over one another as if you were washing them in the sink. Feel free to use a little pressure as you gently rub the palms of your hands, backs of your hands, fingers, and wrists.

Support your right hand with the fingers and palm of the left hand. Gently massage the palm of your right hand with the thumb of your left hand. Massage from the heel of your hand out to the base of your fingers.

Massage the length of each finger. Give the end of each finger a little squeeze.

Thread the fingers of your left hand into the webbing between your fingers and massage the skin between your fingers. Give the space between your index finger and your thumb a little extra love.

Repeat on the other hand.

## Getting Started with Mudras

If meditation and mudras are new to you, I recommend that you start small. Start by meditating for a few minutes at a time and slowly build your "endurance." Be kind and compassionate with yourself when you find your mind jumping from thought to thought. When your attention drifts, and it will, gently bring your awareness back to the mudra, the breath, and the meditation. Know that two minutes of practicing a mudra is better than no minutes practicing a mudra. As the practice becomes more comfortable you can work up to 10, 15, 45, or more minutes of meditation at a time. Eventually, you may choose to practice your mudras twice a day.

One of the great things about mudras is that they can literally be practiced anywhere at any time. Over the course of history, it has been recommended that meditation be practiced at sunrise and sunset. I personally recommend incorporating your mudra and meditation practice into your morning routine before your mind begins to engage with the outside world.

Habit gurus talk about identifying a trigger, or something that happens every day, when you want to create a new habit. For example, if you want to start going to the gym before work, your alarm clock would be the trigger for putting on your workout clothes and gym shoes. When I first began practicing mudras and meditation, I really struggled with making time for meditation. So, I asked myself, "How can I make it easy?" The answer?

Alarm clock goes off. I hit snooze. I stay in bed—but I sit up and find a comfortable seat for meditation. I meditate. When my snooze alarm goes off, my meditation practice is complete. When life gets crazy and doesn't go as planned, I fall back on this same habitual routine. Other trigger examples could be arriving at the office and sitting in your chair, walking in the front door after work, brushing your teeth, sitting at a red light, taking a seat on the Metro, putting the kids to sleep, or even crawling into bed at the end of the day. Identify a trigger and allow that trigger to signal you to begin your mudra practice.

If you find your fingers, hands, wrists, or shoulders getting achy as you practice, take a moment to stretch, or give yourself a massage. Remember, your mudra practice is all about bringing forth more joy, healing, self-care, and balance.

May your journey into the mudras bring you much health, happiness, and joy.

CHAPTER TWO

# Heal and Thrive

I n this chapter you will find 10 mudras to help you thrive by bringing balance and health to your physical body. The mudras included here are meant to help you find relief from stress, pain, fatigue, and burnout. You'll learn to manage and balance the physical elements to nourish and heal your physical body, restore physical strength, and improve digestion and sleep.

## VITALITY AND VIGOR
### Vajra Mudra / Thunderbolt Gesture

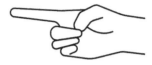

**Chakras:** Root, Sacral, Solar Plexus

**Also good for:** circulatory system health, clarity, concentration, empowerment, motivation, spine health, spiritual awakening

Vajra Mudra and its variations have been practiced for centuries across Asia—from India to South Korea. This mudra is all about increasing vitality and energy. When we're suffering from fatigue or listlessness, this mudra helps us bring vitality, vigor, and enthusiasm to life. It helps us triumph over the 4 p.m. doldrums by sparking the inner fire at our third chakra. The next time you're experiencing the post-lunch "blahs," or that afternoon slump, take a five-minute mudra and meditation break. You'll come back to the task at hand with renewed motivation, passion, and purpose. This mudra is great because you can practice it anytime.

1. With each hand, extend your index fingers out long. Allow your pinky, ring, and middle fingers to curl in gently. Align the fingers of your pinky, ring, and middle fingers, so the sides of your fingernails are touching.
2. Bring your thumbs to touch the side of your middle fingers' fingernail. Rest the backs of your hands on your thighs or knees.
3. Hold for 5 to 15 minutes a day.

## Stoking the Inner Fire Meditation

1. Find a comfortable seat with your pelvis firmly resting on the floor, a cushion, or the edge of a chair. Take a moment or two to move your spine in all directions: Round and arch your back, side bend right and left, and make giant circles with your rib cage. This will help you sit with a long spine and get your blood flowing to clear any stagnant energy in your center.

2. Bring your hands into Vajra Mudra and rest the backs of your hands on your thighs or knees. Close your eyes and take a few rounds of Three-Part Breath (page 15).

3. Now, envision a golden cord flowing down from your third chakra, behind your navel, through the lower chakras, out the base of your spine. This cord continues all the way down through the fertile layer of the Earth's crust, down through its rocky mantle and into its fiery center.

4. Feel the energy of Earth's fiery center flowing up the cord into Manipura, your third chakra. This energy flow nourishes and invigorates you.

5. "See" the wheels of your first, second, and third chakras come alive. They spin brightly in crimson red, vibrant orange, and glowing yellow, respectively. The light at your third chakra grows brighter and brighter. You feel its vibrant energy as heat emanates from your core.

Continued

## Stoking the Inner Fire Meditation   Continued

6. Continue to envision vibrant, golden light flowing up from Earth's core into Manipura. Feel yourself come alive with vitality, vigor, and enthusiasm. Hold your awareness at Manipura for a few minutes, or until you feel complete.
7. Release the imagery and sit in stillness for a few minutes more. Notice how you feel.

# NOURISHMENT AND GUT EASE
## Pushan Mudra / Sun God Gesture

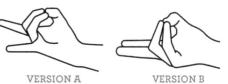

VERSION A          VERSION B

**Chakras:** Root, Solar Plexus

**Also good for:** abundance, energy, immunity, nausea, safe travels, seasickness, workplace meetings, wealth

In Ayurveda, yoga's sister science of holistic wellness, good health relies on healthy digestion. The bacteria in our gut help with digestion, nutrient production, waste elimination, and immune system regulation. Pushan Mudra is named after the Hindu sun god, Pushan, also sometimes called the god of nourishment. In Hindu mythology, Pushan is the supporter and nourisher of Mother Earth, the knower of all animals, and protector of the soul. His name comes from the Sanskrit word *pusyati*, which means "cause to thrive." The Sun's solar energy is associated with our third chakra, our center of personal power and digestion of both food and ideas. Practice Pushan Mudra when your digestive fire is low, you're gassy and bloated, or when your digestive system needs a little TLC.

NOTE: This mudra is asymmetrical and has two versions, one for upper-digestive health and one for lower-digestive health.

**FOR VERSION A, FOR THE HEALTH OF YOUR UPPER DIGESTIVE SYSTEM:**

1. With your left hand, bring your middle and ring fingers to touch your thumb. Your index and pinky fingers are extended long. Your left hand is the same for both versions.
2. With your right hand, bring your index and middle fingers to touch your thumb and extend your ring and pinky fingers.
3. Hold for a minimum of five minutes.

**FOR VERSION B, FOR THE HEALTH OF YOUR LOWER DIGESTIVE SYSTEM:**

1. Position your left hand as indicated for version A.
2. With your right hand, bring your ring and pinky fingers to touch the tip of your thumb and extend your index and middle fingers out long.
3. Hold for a minimum of five minutes.

## Samana Vayu Meditation

Samana Vayu is the integrating and balancing vayu. It draws prana toward the center and aids digestion of food, information, and thoughts.

1. Find a comfortable seat and assume either variation of Pushan Mudra.
2. Begin by cultivating a soft Ujjayi breath, which helps regulate the flow of your inhale and exhale and create heat within the body. To practice

Ujjayi, breathe in and out through your nose, creating a gentle constriction in the back of your throat. Hear your breath as it creates an audible, oceanic sound.

3. Begin to lengthen each inhale and exhale to four or five counts each. When you exhale, become aware of your navel drawing in toward your spine. Maintain a gentle Ujjayi breath throughout the meditation.

4. Bring your awareness to the crown of your head. As you inhale, imagine a warm white light flowing into the crown of your head and down to your navel center. As you exhale, envision the warm white light flowing out from your navel center to fill your entire body with prana—energy. With each inhale, warm white light flows from your crown to your navel. Each exhale sees warm white light flow from your navel out into the field of your body.

5. With each cycle of breath, repeat one, or all, of the following mantras:

I choose foods that nourish my well-being.

I accept nourishment with ease and grace.

I am healthy and thriving.

## STRESS RELEASE AND RELIEF
### Sukham Mudra / Delight Gesture

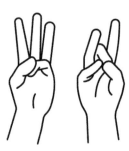

**Chakras:** Root, Sacral, Throat

**Also good for:** creating flow and adaptability, letting go of what no longer serves us

In the *Yoga Sutras of Patanjali*, Patanjali says, "Sthira-sukham asanam," or "Our seat should be both steady and easeful." This sutra, however, applies not only to our meditation practice, but also life as a whole. For many of us, we're overscheduled, overtasked, overstimulated, exhausted, burned-out, stressed out, and no longer connected to the cycles and rhythms of nature. Raise your hand if you can relate! Chronic stress is linked to mental health issues, cardiovascular disease, and gastrointestinal disorders. Now is the time to take charge of your joy and happiness and ask for the help you need. Sukham is all about creating ease, happiness, harmony, flow, and joy. It's about creating time to slow down and get present with our essence, with our truth.

Practice Sukham Mudra when life feels tied to the clock, you're burning the candle at both ends, and you're feeling stressed and overwhelmed.

1. With your right hand, bring your middle and pinky fingers to touch the tip of your thumb and extend your ring and index fingers straight.

2. With your left hand, press your thumb over the top of your pinky fingernail and extend the index, middle, and ring fingers out straight.
3. Practice for a few minutes at a time to combat stress and exhaustion.

## Manifest Joy Meditation

1. Clear 20 to 30 minutes in your schedule. Go outside to a favorite park, trail, river, lake, beach, garden, or other available spot. Find a place where you will be comfortable and undisturbed. For this meditation, you can sit, lie down, or even walk at a slow and mindful pace.
2. Bring your hands into Sukham Mudra and close your eyes or find a soft gaze.
3. Take a few full belly breaths—in through your nose and out through your mouth. On each inhale, invite vibrant energy in and with each exhale, release stress, worry, to-do lists, etc. Take as many rounds of breaths as necessary.
4. Now bring your mind's eye to an easeful day going about your usual tasks. What does it look like? What happens or doesn't happen? Who is there? Is there time to do a favorite activity? Is there time to be still? How does it feel when everything flows easefully? Savor the ease for 5 to 10 minutes.

Continued

## Manifest Joy Meditation    Continued

5. Sukham Mudra works with the elements of earth (structure and stability), water (flow and release), and ether (lightness) and the root, sacral, and throat chakras. In your journal, reflect on which of these three elements, or chakras, could use a little extra attention. Do you need more structure? More flexibility and flow? Or more lightness? Write down three steps you can take to manifest more joy in your life.

## PASSION AND ENERGY
### Linga Mudra / Gesture of the Divine Masculine

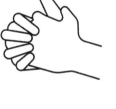

**Chakras:** Root, Solar Plexus

**Also good for:** concentration, depression, men's health, metabolism, weight loss, willpower

Linga Mudra is associated with the energy of the Divine masculine and of Shiva, or cosmic consciousness. We all have both the Divine masculine and the Divine feminine within us. When we are aligned with the Divine masculine, we're confident, courageous, passionate, and energetic. Linga Mudra can be practiced when we're feeling lethargic, our metabolism is slow, and we are unmotivated. Linga Mudra increases pitta in the body, which is associated with the fire and water elements. By increasing pitta, we can increase our metabolism, digestive fire, and our ability to get things done. Practice Linga Mudra when you have a big task coming up that will require lots of energy, enthusiasm, and focus.

1. Bring your hands to touch and interlace your fingers with your left index finger over the top of your right index finger.
2. Extend your right thumb upward, as if you were hitchhiking. Wrap the index finger and thumb of your left hand around the base of your right thumb.
3. Hold the mudra for 15 to 45 minutes with your hands in front of your navel.

## Tratak Meditation

For this meditation, you will need a candle or flame to focus your eyes on. If you don't have a candle available, use an uplifting image instead.

1. Place the candle flame a few feet in front of you, at eye level or slightly lower.
2. Bring the palms of your hands in front of you and rub them together vigorously until they become warm. Gently place the palms over your eyes and hold them there until the heat dissipates. Repeat two more times.
3. Bring your hands into Linga Mudra. Try to keep the mudra in front of your navel throughout the meditation. If your arms become tired, rest your hands in your lap with the right thumb still upright.
4. Bring your soft eye gaze to the candle flame. Hold your gaze on the flame without blinking and without strain. When your eyes begin to water or become strained, close your eyes and hold the vision of the candle flame with your eyes closed.
5. When you can no longer "see" the candle flame with your eyes closed, open your eyes and begin again. Repeat this meditation for up to 10 minutes.
6. Once you finish, release the mudra and bring the palms of your hands to touch again. Rub your palms together vigorously and place them over your eyes. Repeat as necessary.

# EAR HEALTH AND DEEP LISTENING
## Shunya Mudra / Gesture of the Void

**Chakras:** Throat

**Also good for:** jet lag, motion sickness

Shunya Mudra has been traditionally practiced to bring health to the ears, in particular to those who experience earache, tinnitus, or hearing issues.

Shunya Mudra works with the ether element by minimizing its excess. This mudra is particularly helpful for those who travel a lot and may help equalize your ears. The act of travel also takes us away from our roots and can leave us feeling ungrounded, with our head stuck in the clouds. If you're feeling "spacey" or "stuck in your head," this mudra can help bring you down to Earth.

My favorite application of this mudra is for deep listening, which is listening with an open mind. It is listening with our full presence without judgment, expectation, or control. When we listen deeply, we do not think about how we will reply or how right or wrong the person speaking is. We listen with curiosity. We witness fully. Deep listening encourages open and honest dialogue. Practice Shunya Mudra for presence and groundedness, inner and outer listening, and cultivating empathy.

1. Shunya Mudra should be practiced in a comfortable seated position and in a quiet, peaceful location.
2. With each hand, bring the tip of the middle finger to the base of the thumb and then fold the thumb over the middle finger. The other fingers are extended long.
3. Practice up to 45 minutes per day.

## Deep Listening Meditation

1. Find a comfortable seat and close your eyes. Bring your awareness to your sense of hearing. Become aware of the most distant sounds you hear: the sounds of traffic, a plane flying overhead, your neighbors chatting, the hum of the washing machine in the next room. Follow the distant sounds and notice the space between the sounds. Notice the moments of quiet.
2. Invite your awareness to nearer sounds: the sound of a fan, the buzz of electricity, your pup's breathing. Stay with each sound for a moment and then allow your awareness to shift to another sound. Become aware of the pauses between sounds.
3. Now invite your awareness to the sounds within your physical body: the sound of your breath, the movement of your clothes, the rumble of digestion, the sacred rhythm of your heart, the beat of your pulse within

your ears. Again, stay with each sound for a few moments. Notice the moments of quiet.

4. Finally, bring your awareness to the sounds of your own thoughts. Follow each thought for a moment and then release it. Meet your thoughts as they arise with no judgment—only kindness and compassion. Notice the space between one thought and the next. Know that the gaps between thoughts will lengthen with practice and patience.

# HEALTHY HANDS: FLEXIBILITY

Hand, wrist, and finger flexibility is often overlooked, but it's important for our overall well-being. You can easily incorporate this short stretching sequence into your day.

1. Bring the palms of your hands to touch and interlace your fingers. Move your hands in "figure eights" a few times in each direction. This will help loosen your wrists and forearms.
2. Extend your arms out to the side. Splay your fingers wide and then make fists. Do this quickly, as if your hands were strobe lights.
3. Now it's time to stretch those digits. Extend your right arm in front of you with your fingertips pointing down. With your left hand, take hold of your right pinky finger and gently pull it back toward you until you feel a gentle stretch. Repeat this stretch for each finger. Switch hands.
4. Interlace the fingers of your hands again. This time, turn the palms away from you and stretch your arms forward while you press out through the palms of your hands. Pause here for a moment and then take your arms overhead. Bring your open palms to the back of your head, take your elbows wide, and lift your chest. Breathe deeply.

## HEALING ENERGY AND PAIN MANAGEMENT
### Mukula Mudra / Lotus Bud Gesture

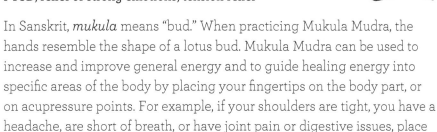

**Chakras:** Heart, Root, Sacral, Solar Plexus

**Also good for:** calm, concentration, PTSD, relief of strong emotions, tension relief

In Sanskrit, *mukula* means "bud." When practicing Mukula Mudra, the hands resemble the shape of a lotus bud. Mukula Mudra can be used to increase and improve general energy and to guide healing energy into specific areas of the body by placing your fingertips on the body part, or on acupressure points. For example, if your shoulders are tight, you have a headache, are short of breath, or have joint pain or digestive issues, place the tips of your fingers on these parts of your body.

Mukula Mudra can also be combined with a therapeutic technique created by Gary Craig called Emotional Freedom Techniques (EFT), sometimes simply called "tapping." A study by Dr. Dawson Church published in the journal *Traumatology* found that EFT is an effective therapy for improving symptoms of PTSD. The study found that 86 percent of study participants dropped below the clinical threshold for PTSD after just six sessions. The therapy is now an accepted treatment by the United States Department of Veterans Affairs and free resources are available online. Emotional Freedom Techniques involve identifying the issue and adding a positive statement of self-acceptance while tapping a series of points along the meridian lines of the body, which are energetic lines used in traditional Chinese medicine and acupuncture. There is much overlap between the meridian lines of Chinese medicine and the nadis of yoga and Ayurveda. An example of your positive statement could be "Even though my lower back aches, I find ease and relief from tension and discomfort."

1. To practice Mukula Mudra, bring the tips of your fingers to the tip of your thumb.
2. For general energy, rest the backs of your hands on your thighs or knees.
3. For targeted energy healing or pain relief, point your fingertips at the body parts that need extra TLC.
4. Hold for 5 to 30 minutes, or as needed.

## Pain Relief Meditation

1. Come into a comfortable seated posture and bring your hands into Mukula Mudra.
2. Sit quietly for a moment and check in with your physical body. Become aware of any places of tension, tightness, pain, or restriction.
3. Begin to deepen your breath and send your breath into these tight, restricted places.

4. Choose one tense or painful place on your body and bring your fingertips to this spot. Envision healing, rejuvenating energy, prana, flowing from your fingertips into this spot.

5. You may even choose to incorporate a statement like the one just noted: "Even though my shoulders are tense and painful now, I know one day I will no longer experience this pain."

6. When you're ready, move your awareness to another part of your body that needs extra healing attention. Bring your fingers, in Mukula Mudra, to this new body part and again envision healing, vibrant energy flowing out of your fingertips back into your body. Keep breathing slowly and deeply. You may use the same mantra or create a new one.

7. Practice this for 15 to 20 minutes, working your way around your body, releasing tension and tightness as you go.

## PHYSICAL STRENGTH
### Prithvi Mudra / Earth Gesture

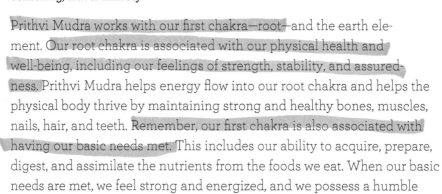

**Chakras:** Root

**Also good for:** digestion, emotional balance, fatigue relief, general anxiety, grounding and centering, travel anxiety

Prithvi Mudra works with our first chakra—root—and the earth element. Our root chakra is associated with our physical health and well-being, including our feelings of strength, stability, and assuredness. Prithvi Mudra helps energy flow into our root chakra and helps the physical body thrive by maintaining strong and healthy bones, muscles, nails, hair, and teeth. Remember, our first chakra is also associated with having our basic needs met. This includes our ability to acquire, prepare, digest, and assimilate the nutrients from the foods we eat. When our basic needs are met, we feel strong and energized, and we possess a humble confidence.

If you're experiencing a time of great transition, such as a big move, career change, or upcoming event that makes you feel weak in the knees, practice Prithvi Mudra anytime you can—in meditation, at the office, walking around town, or on your commute.

1. On each hand, bring the tip of your ring finger to the tip of your thumb and extend your index, middle, and pinky fingers out long. Point your fingertips down toward the ground.
2. Practice for up to 15 minutes at a time.

## Walking Meditation

1. Find a place where you can walk barefoot; this could be in your home, yard, a park, garden, or beach, for example.
2. Take your shoes off, stand tall, and bring your hands into Prithvi Mudra with your fingers pointing down.
3. Close your eyes. If you feel unbalanced with your eyes closed, keep them open, or take a comfortable seat.
4. Position your feet hip-width apart with your toes pointing forward. Move your attention to the soles of your feet. Ground down through the four corners of each foot: the inner and outer heel, the big toe ball mound, and the little toe ball mound. Lift your toes up, splay them wide, and try to place them back down one at a time. Observe the subtle lift through the arches of your feet.
5. Feel the texture and temperature of the ground beneath you.

Continued

## Walking Meditation   Continued

6. Allow your eyes to flutter open and maintain a soft downward gaze. Slowly step forward with your right foot, being mindful of the engagement of the muscles in your legs, hips, and core as your leg lifts. Notice your left foot as the weight shifts and the heel lifts. Feel the strength in your calf, arches, and toes as the left foot pushes off. The right foot steps down, heel to toe. Begin to walk in this manner. Step slowly and mindfully. Be fully aware of your feet connecting to the Earth. With each step, be aware of the ground beneath you providing stability and support.

7. Take your time. Walk in this manner for 10 to 30 minutes.

## CLEANSE AND RELEASE
### Apana Mudra / Cleansing Gesture

**Chakras:** Root, Sacral, Solar Plexus, Throat

**Also good for:** arthritis, clearing out emotional baggage, creative energy, menstruation, new beginnings, skin health, urinary health

Apana is the energy of cleansing and clearing. It is a downward and outward flowing energy that governs our ability to release and let go of physical waste as well as emotional baggage. Apana Mudra is practiced to bring health to the organs between our navel and perineum and aid our ability to move toxins and waste down and out. If you experience constipation or indigestion, practice Apana Mudra for up to 30 minutes.

In addition to helping release physical waste from the body, this mudra can help clear the emotional waste we carry around day in and day out. Practice this mudra when you're ready to release negative emotions, grudges, and judgments, and create more serenity, balance, and harmony.

Apana Mudra works with the earth element and is an excellent mudra to practice outdoors, surrounded by nature.

1. Using just one hand, or both hands, bring the tips of your middle and ring fingers to touch the tip of your thumb. Extend your pinky and index fingers out long.
2. Practice up to three times per day, for a total of 30 to 45 minutes.

## Sacred Garden Meditation

1. You can practice this meditation indoors or outdoors in a comfortable seat. Perhaps sit in Vajrasana, which is a kneeling yoga posture in which you're seated on your heels.
2. Close your eyes and take a moment to center yourself. Rock your head side to side. Take a couple of shoulder circles and then settle into stillness. Bring one or both hands into Apana Mudra.
3. Imagine you are sitting in a lush, green garden surrounded by ancient shade trees with roots reaching deep down into the Earth and wide, sweeping branches that extend up toward the heavens. The garden is rich with life. It is a sacred cocoon for you and all the beings within it. The flowers are in bloom. Butterflies, dragonflies, and honeybees flit about. Hummingbirds drink rich nectar from the flowers and birds gently splash in a nearby stream. You experience an effortless sense of balance, peace, and harmony.

4. You reach down and put your hands into the fertile Earth. You feel the moistness of the soil as it gently crumbles and falls through your fingers. You know that here, within the safety of this fertile garden, there is no need to hold on tightly to that which no longer serves you. The soil willingly receives the residue left behind from both physical toxins and emotional baggage and turns them into fertile compost. With each exhale breath, release holding, release grasping, release negativity.
5. You've just released all that doesn't serve you, both physical and emotional. Take a moment to savor this release. Ask yourself what would nourish you most right now.
6. Take a moment to sit quietly.

## BETTER NIGHT'S SLEEP
### Shakti Mudra /
### Gesture of the Divine Feminine

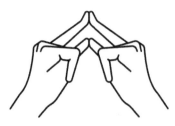

**Chakras:** Sacral

**Also good for:** calming the nervous system, improving personal power, relief from menstrual cramps, sexual health, women's health

Shakti Mudra is one of my favorite mudras for stress- and anxiety-related insomnia. When my mind is spinning and I can't fall asleep, Shakti Mudra is one of my go-to practices. If you've had a long day at work or you're under a lot of outside pressure to "get things done," Shakti Mudra can help you feel empowered and in control of the situation. It also relieves those nagging feelings of anxiety lurking in the shadows. When you're struggling to get good, quality sleep, practice Shakti Mudra for 10 to 15 minutes before bed with a slow, deep breath. It will help you calm your nervous system and prepare you for a better night's sleep.

This mudra is also associated with our sacral chakra and it helps us embrace our creativity and artistic expression. It helps us embody fluidity, flow, and flexibility. If you're working on a fun, creative project, Shakti Mudra can help get your creative juices flowing.

1. For Shakti Mudra, fold the thumb of each hand into the palm and then fold the index finger and middle finger over the top of each thumb. Extend your ring and pinky fingers out long and bring the tips of your right and left ring and pinky fingers to touch.
2. Practice three times a day for 15 minutes at a time.

## Honoring the Divine Feminine Meditation

1. Find a comfortable seated position. Close your eyes and bring your awareness to your breath.
2. Bring your hands into Shakti Mudra. Begin your practice with Three-Part Breathing (page 15) and stay with this pranayama for a few minutes until you feel calm and centered.
3. As you follow your breath, bring your awareness to your breathing diaphragm. Take a moment to experience the rise and fall of your breathing diaphragm as you exhale and inhale.
4. Now bring awareness to your pelvic floor, also sometimes called your pelvic diaphragm. Experience the subtle influence of your breath here. Notice that on inhale your pelvic floor diaphragm moves down and, on exhale, it lifts. Both diaphragms move in unison.
5. If you're preparing for bed, stay here and witness the breath while practicing the mudra.

Continued

6. If you are seeking help with accessing your Divine feminine, or creative expression, chant the following mantra: "Hrim Shrim Klim Parameshwari Swaha" (pronounced, *hreem shreem kleem pah-rahm-esh-wah-ree swa-ha*), which translates to "Salutations to the Supreme Feminine. May that abundant principle that hides the nature of ultimate reality be attracted to me." In addition, this mantra helps us see the world as it really is and helps us cultivate feelings of positivity and abundance. Repeat this mantra 27, 54, or 108 times (108 is a sacred number in yoga and Ayurveda and is divisible by 27 and 54).

## RADIANT, FLOWING BEAUTY
### Varuna Mudra /
### Gesture of the God of Water

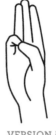 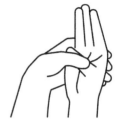

VERSION A    VERSION B

**Chakras:** Sacral

**Also good for:** flexibility, memory, sexual health, skin health

Varuna is one of the oldest Vedic deities. In modern Hinduism, he is considered the god of the West and ruler and protector of the oceans, rivers, aquatic animals, and the rains. Varuna Mudra helps us regulate the water element in our physical body. This mudra has two versions: one to *increase* the water element and one to *decrease* the water element. We practice Varuna Mudra (version A) when we are feeling dried out, lackluster, rigid, and achy. Varuna Mudra bathes our second chakra, reproductive organs, and skin in nourishing prana. This mudra can help restore our youthful, radiant glow. Varuna Mudra, version B, reduces the water element in our body, which can be used if you were experiencing bloating, edema, congestion, or excess mucus.

FOR VERSION A, TO *INCREASE* THE WATER ELEMENT IN THE BODY:

1. On each hand, bring the tip of your pinky finger to the tip of your thumb. Extend your other fingers out straight.
2. Practice for up to 45 minutes per day.

**FOR VERSION B, TO *REDUCE* THE WATER ELEMENT IN THE BODY:**

1. Bring your right pinky finger to the base of your right thumb and fold your thumb over the top of your pinky finger. Your index, middle, and ring fingers extend straight out.
2. Rest your right hand in the palm of your left hand and wrap your left thumb over the top of your right thumb. Apply gentle pressure.
3. Practice for up to 45 minutes per day.

## Water Meditation

1. For this meditation, use Varuna Mudra, version A.
2. Lie on your back. Wiggle around a bit and get comfortable. If you have an achy lower back, place a bolster, cushion, or pillow underneath your knees. With the knees supported, your lower back will relax and soften into the support beneath you. You're now in a restorative yoga pose that resembles a mountain brook—your body like the polished stones in a creek.
3. Close your eyes and envision your body surrounded by cool, gently flowing water.
4. Envision water flowing around and over your body. Become aware of its pauses and eddies, and where the water flows more briskly.

5. Envision this water washing away impurities, tension, worries. It washes away self-doubt, circular thinking, and stress.
6. And, just like water flowing over stones or through a river gorge, it smooths your edges, it softens your worry lines and mellows your temper, showing you the path of least resistance.
7. As it clears out your stress, it fills you with the essence of flow, the essence of ease.
8. The water continues to flow over your body and through your body. It nourishes every cell.
9. Envision the stream water balancing the water element in your physical body.
10. Stay with this visualization for the next 5 to 10 minutes.
11. This same meditation can be practiced, seated, for version B. To hold version B on your back is not as comfortable as version A.

# CHAPTER THREE

# Energize and Balance

T his chapter focuses on bringing balance and healing to matters of energy and spirituality. You will find mudras and meditations to help guide you on your spiritual journey. These mudras will help you find clarity and confidence as you move along your path of transformation with authenticity and integrity.

## OVERCOME OBSTACLES
### Ganesha Mudra /
### Remover of Obstacles Gesture

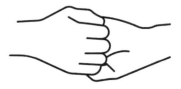

**Chakras:** Heart, Solar Plexus

**Also good for:** acceptance, confidence, courage, good health, happiness, inner wisdom, love, perseverance, sacrifice

Ganesha, known as the elephant god, is the remover of obstacles. His statues are commonplace in homes, temples, and gathering places wherever Hinduism is practiced. You can practice Ganesha Mudra to clear both physical and spiritual obstacles from your path. Ganesha helps us transcend maya, the obstacle of illusion, and he blesses our endeavors. Ganesha and this mudra teach us to tap into our inner wisdom by listening deeply and seeing beyond the illusory.

If you're beginning a new project, whether personal, spiritual, or professional, practice Ganesha Mudra each morning to bless and honor the beginning of a new day, free of obstacles. When life's challenges feel overwhelming, practice Ganesha Mudra and you may find the alternative solutions you seek. Ganesha teaches us to work around our problems instead of blasting through them with the force of dynamite. I like to practice Ganesha Mudra seated, but it can be a great addition to any asana practice and easily incorporated into many poses like Warrior 1, Tree pose, or Chair pose.

1. Bring your hands in front of your heart space. Turn your left palm away from you and your right palm toward you. Bend the fingers of each hand and hook them together.
2. Maintain the mudra. While you inhale, pull your elbows away from one another. You will feel tension between the hands increase and the muscles around your arms and shoulders engage. Relax as you exhale.
3. Repeat 10 to 15 times.

### Ganesha Bhakti Meditation

1. Bhakti is a path of devotion and love toward a personal deity. In Sanskrit, bhakti means faith, love, devotion, worship, and a fondness for. This path of yoga requires participation, devotion, and love. One way to practice bhakti yoga is by chanting. In this meditation, we will explore a chant to Ganesha as we practice Ganesha Mudra.
2. Find a comfortable seated position and bring your hands into Ganesha Mudra. In this meditation, feel free to switch the clasp of your hands as needed.

Continued

3. Take three cleansing rounds of breath—in through your nose and out through your mouth. When you exhale, release physical, mental, and emotional resistance.

4. The chant you will use is "Om Gam Ganapataye Namaha" (pronounced *ohm gahm gah-nah-paht-ah-yeh nah-mah-hah*), and, essentially, means "I offer my salutations and I bow to Lord Ganesha, the remover of obstacles." Repeat this chant 27, 54, or 108 times either out loud or internally (108 is a sacred number in yoga and Ayurveda, and 108 is divisible by 27 and 54).

5. If chanting to Ganesha does not resonate with you, try one of the following affirmations:

I overcome obstacles with ease and grace.

My path is blessed by _____.

I see clearly and act with love, courage, and confidence.

## COURAGE AND CONFIDENCE
### Pran Mudra / Energy Seal

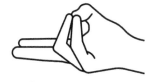

**Chakras:** Heart, Root, Solar Plexus, Third Eye, Throat

**Also good for:** digestion, improving concentration, inner fire, self-healing, uplifting

Pran Vayu is the energy flowing between the head and the heart. Pran Mudra grounds the energy of Pran Vayu and provides a sense of aliveness and vitality. When our physical body is healthy and prana is flowing, we feel strong, confident, and courageous. This mudra amplifies these qualities and gives us the strength, endurance, and willpower to see things through. We have abundant energy and the confidence to step outside our comfort zone and try something new. I practice Pran Mudra when I need to shift out of a cycle of fear and doubt and into a mind-set of positivity and courage.

Pran Mudra is also a fantastic mudra to practice after lunch. It fans the flames of our digestive fire and helps us feel light and vibrant, instead of heavy and lethargic. Cain Carroll, author of *Mudras of Yoga*, an amazing mudra resource, teaches that Pran Mudra "activates the body's self-healing potential . . . and decreases the body's susceptibility to injury and disease." I'm all for living a happy, healthy, vibrant life—and I'm sure you are, too.

1. On each hand, extend your index and middle fingers out long. Bend your ring and pinky fingers and bring the pads of your thumbs to cover their fingernails.
2. Rest the backs of your hands on your thighs or knees, or extend your arms straight out to the side at shoulder height. This is an excellent mudra to incorporate into yoga poses such as Warrior II, Goddess pose, or Triangle pose.
3. If you're practicing Pran Mudra in a seated posture, you may hold the mudra for 5 to 45 minutes.

## Pran Vayu Meditation

1. Find a comfortable seated position. Bring your hands into Pran Mudra and bring the backs of your hands to your thighs and knees.
2. Guide your awareness to your breath in your head and heart space. Balance the length of your inhale and exhale, and experience your breath fully.
3. On your inhale, envision the white light of prana pouring in though the five gates of your senses: eyes, ears, nose, mouth, and skin. This white light flows toward your third eye.
4. Pause and retain your breath for a moment as you envision a glowing ball of white light at your third eye.

5. With your exhale, witness the flow of prana out through the gates of your five senses.
6. Witness the flow of prana as it flows in and out through the five gates of your senses.
7. Each cycle of breath bathes your brain in pranic energy. Each cycle of breath rejuvenates your body and mind and nourishes your being.
8. Sit quietly and bask in this radiance. Stay with this visualization for 10 to 15 minutes.

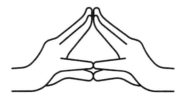

## CONCENTRATION
### Hakini Mudra /
### Third Eye Goddess Gesture

**Chakras:** Crown, Heart, Root, Sacral, Solar Plexus, Third Eye, Throat

**Also good for:** cooperation, communication between the right and left hemispheres of the brain, fresh ideas, improving and deepening respiration, knowledge of the truth and of nonduality, memory, problem-solving

You've likely seen Hakini Mudra practiced in "unlikely" places—like in the office conference room, during a board meeting, or even at a sporting event. We naturally take this mudra when we're processing incoming information or seeking a solution to a problem. Hakini Mudra is also great if you've lost your train of thought. If you find yourself circling back to the same old ideas, Hakini Mudra is like a breath of fresh air as it invites us to see the big picture from a different point of view.

1. This mudra is best practiced in a seated position. Bring the tips of your fingers of your right hand to meet the tips of your fingers of your left hand. The palms of the hands are pulled away from one another.
2. I've found the best results when I bring the mudra in front of my navel for matters of the ego; in front of my heart for matters of the heart; or in front of my third eye for intuition, insight, and broadened awareness.
3. Hold for 5 to 45 minutes.

1. Hakini Mudra is often practiced with the specific breathing technique taught here.

2. Bring your hands into Hakini Mudra and place your hands at the navel, heart, or third eye. Close your eyes. If you're trying to find solutions to a specific question or challenge, ask your higher self for insight and guidance now.

3. Shift your awareness to your breath. Inhale and press your tongue to the roof of your mouth behind your teeth; when you exhale, relax your tongue. Practice 5 to 10 times.

4. Bring your awareness to your third eye. Hold your awareness here for a moment and experience your third eye without distraction.

5. Shift your awareness out beyond the tip of your nose. Pause here for another moment.

6. Invite your awareness to flow outward to your immediate surroundings. Hold the vision of your nearest surroundings at your third eye.

7. Move your awareness out a little further. Within your third-eye space, see yourself, see your home, see your city, see your state, province, and country.

8. Within your mind's eye, see Earth in its entirety. Pause here and experience it fully.

Continued

9. Now your awareness moves out to into Space. Experience the vastness of Space with a sense of calm, clarity, and connection. Perhaps it is here you will find the answer to your question.

10. Experience each layer fully as you gently bring your awareness back to the third eye, one layer at a time. Hold your awareness at your third eye for a few minutes longer.

## DIVINE WISDOM
### Jnana Mudra / Knowledge Gesture

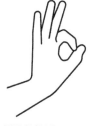

VERSION A    VERSION B

**Chakras:** Crown, Heart, Root, Solar Plexus, Third Eye

**Also good for:** bringing unity, calming, clearing the mind, devotion, enhancing consciousness, harmony, intuition, peace, relieving insomnia and tiredness

Jnana Mudra is one of the most recognizable mudras in all of yoga. It is one of the most iconic mudras of meditation practitioners worldwide and it has been depicted widely in images of deities and pop culture alike.

This was the very first mudra I learned. In this mudra, the index finger represents the individual ego, or individual consciousness, and the thumb represents cosmic consciousness, or Divine wisdom. In version A, you *unite the individual consciousness* with the universal consciousness. In version B, you *surrender the ego* to the Divine by bringing the thumb over the top of the index finger.

Jnana Mudra is best practiced in meditation, when you would like to cultivate a sense of unity and harmony, or when you're seeking wisdom from a higher source.

**FOR VERSION A, TO *UNITE THE INDIVIDUAL CONSCIOUSNESS* WITH THE UNIVERSAL CONSCIOUSNESS:**

1. Find a comfortable seat. On each hand, bring the tip of your index finger to the tip of your thumb and extend your other fingers.
2. Hold for a minimum of five minutes; this can be done for the entirety of your meditation practice.

**FOR VERSION B, TO *SURRENDER THE EGO* TO THE DIVINE:**

1. Find a comfortable seat. On each hand, bring the pad of your thumb over the nail of your index finger. The remaining fingers extend long.
2. Turn the palms down for a feeling of groundedness; turn your palms upward in a gesture of receptivity for a feeling of lightness.
3. You may also bring the mudra with your right hand in front of your heart space.
4. Hold for a minimum of five minutes; this can be done for the entirety of your meditation practice.

## Mindfulness Meditation

Mindfulness meditation teaches us to listen deeply and compassionately to the thoughts and chatter of our own mind, so we may be equally present with others.

1. Come into a comfortable seated position and bring your hands into Jnana Mudra. Turn the palms of your hands down if it is the end of the day, or you're in need of some grounding. If it's morning, or you need a little extra energy to get through your day, turn your palms up.

2. Close your eyes and notice your breath as it flows in through the nostrils, down the back of the throat, and into the lungs. Follow your breath as it leaves the lungs, flows up through the throat, out the nostrils, and across the upper lip. Witness your breath for 5 to 10 breath cycles.

3. Release awareness of your breath and sit quietly. Notice anything that draws your attention—this could be thoughts, sounds, smells, or other sensations.

4. Meet whatever comes into your awareness with kindness and compassion.

5. Sit quietly and notice thoughts and sensations drifting in and out of your awareness without becoming attached. Witness the ebb and flow of your awareness.

6. Stay with this meditation for 10 to 15 minutes. Increase the length of this meditation practice gradually and incrementally.

## INTENTION AND MANIFESTATION
Bija Mudra / Seed Seal

**Chakras:** Crown, Heart, Root, Sacral,
Solar Plexus, Third Eye, Throat

**Also good for:** authenticity, faith, guidance, inner truth

Bija Mudra, or seed seal, is one of my favorite mudras. This powerful mudra helps us receive the gifts of our intuition and inner knowing. It exposes our deepest desires and provides us with the faith, trust, and patience to put those desires into action. This mudra is most powerful during New Moon, Winter Solstice, Spring Equinox, and Beltane rituals. These moments, during the cycles of the moon and seasons, are potent opportunities to plant the seeds of your intentions.

1. I find this mudra most potent when practiced in a seated posture with the hands at heart center.
2. Bring the palms of your hands to touch in front of your heart space. Keep your fingertips, the inner and outer edges of your hands, and the heels of your hands touching as you create a small space between your palms. Your hands will form the shape of a seed.
3. Practice Bija Mudra for 10 to 30 minutes.

## Seed Meditation

1. For this meditation, you will work with what is called a *sankalpa*. A sankalpa is a resolve or intention; for the purpose of this exercise, your sankalpa will be a positive statement or affirmation. Here are a few examples:

I am guided by Divine love.

I am the witness.

I am limitless.

I trust my intuition.

I trust my inner guide to give me the answers I need.

2. Come into a comfortable seated position. Bring your hands into Bija Mudra at your heart center.
3. Close your eyes and witness your breath for a few moments.
4. Now shift your awareness to the sacred rhythm of your heartbeat within your chest.
5. Imagine yourself standing at the edge of a dense, emerald green forest. The forest is behind you. In front of you is an expansive meadow of wildflowers. Across the meadow you see a beautiful, leafy tree.
6. You leave the shade of the forest, step into the meadow, and walk toward the tree. You reach the tree and stand underneath its leafy branches. Sunlight peeks through and dances across your skin.

Continued

7. In the trunk of the tree there is a small hole. Within the hole you see a glowing, perfectly formed seed. You reach in and pick up the seed. Rolling the seed in your hands, you see an inscription. Your sankalpa is written on this seed.

8. You take a seat in the cool shade of the tree and hold the seed gently as a sacred object. You bring the seed close to your heart. Know that this intention resides safely within.

9. Now repeat your sankalpa three times quietly and internally to yourself.

10. Hold this sacred seed in front of your heart for as long as you desire.

# HEALTHY HANDS: STRENGTH

Strong hands and fingers don't just make opening pickle jars easier; they make practicing mudras easier, too. Here we'll explore a few exercises to improve the strength in your hands. These exercises are especially beneficial for those with arthritis or carpal tunnel.

**Warm up:** With the palms of your hands open, curl one finger at a time in toward the center of your palm. Do this two to three times per finger.

**Lateral movements:** With your palms open and fingers extended long, one at a time, move your fingers side to side. Really articulate each movement. Repeat two to three times per finger.

**Fists:** Begin with your palms open, fingers extended long and close together. Begin to curl your fingers in. Articulate through your knuckles as best you can. Uncurl just as mindfully. Repeat 10 times.

**Grip strength #1:** Place a towel, sponge, stress ball, or other soft ball in the palm of your hand and squeeze it. Hold for 10 to 20 seconds. Repeat 5 to 10 times.

**Additional ways to improve hand strength:** Practice arm balances, learn hasta bandha, and carry your heavy grocery bags out to the car instead of pushing them in the cart.

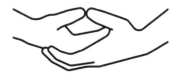

**Chakras:** Crown, Solar Plexus, Third Eye

**Also good for:** concentration, feelings of comfort, safety, and being held, general healing and healing emotional trauma, harmony, inspiration, memory, mindfulness, optimism, spiritual awakening, stress relief

Dhyana is the most prominent mudra in Buddhism and it is believed that Gautama Buddha practiced this mudra in the moment of his enlightenment. In Sanskrit, *dhyana* means meditation. In the beginning stages of meditation, we are often practicing dharana, or focused awareness. As we continue our meditation practice, we may reach the state of dhyana, or union with the object of our meditation. Practicing Dhyana Mudra can help us reach this state of absorption.

Whether you've been practicing meditation for a long time or it's a new practice, you will benefit from Dhyana Mudra. This mudra helps us find calm in chaos and helps us experience more peace, contentment, and connection in our relationships with others, our self, and the Universe.

Dhyana Mudra unites the Divine masculine and feminine within us. The right hand represents the masculine and the left hand represents the feminine. The right hand also sometimes represents enlightenment and truth, whereas the left hand sometimes represents *maya*, or illusion.

With the right hand over the left hand, this mudra represents the growth one experiences on a spiritual journey as its shifts from a state of illusion to a state of enlightenment.

1. In a comfortable seat, rest your left hand in your lap with your palm facing up. Place the back of your right in the palm of your left hand.
2. Bring the tips of your thumbs to touch.
3. Hold for a minimum of five minutes; this can be done for the entirety of your meditation practice.

## So Hum Meditation

Dhyana Mudra is a beautiful and simple mudra; for this meditation we will pair Dhyana Mudra with an equally beautiful and simple mantra: "So Hum." In Sanskrit, *So Hum* means "I am that." So = I am; Hum = that, referring to all of creation and the interconnectedness of all things.

1. This meditation, mudra, and mantra combination is best practiced seated in a quiet location.
2. Sit tall with your rib cage stacked over your pelvis. Find length from the base of your spine out through the crown of your head.
3. Bring your hands into Dhyana Mudra and close your eyes.

Continued

4. Follow the rise and fall of your breath. As you inhale, hear the sound "so"; as you exhale, hear the sound "hum."
5. As you inhale, fill with the expansiveness of the Universe. You are one with the Universe. You are nourished and supported by the Universe.
6. As you exhale, your breath flows outward, mixing into the flow of the Universe. Your breath nourishes the Universe.
7. Experience your breath as whole and complete. It is one with the flow of the Universe.
8. Stay with this meditation for 5 to 15 minutes.

## AUTHENTICITY
### Dharmachakra Mudra / Wheel of Dharma Seal

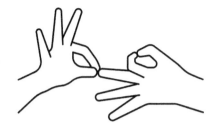

**Chakras:** Heart, Throat

**Also good for:** accessing the wisdom of the heart, calm, creating a continuous flow of prana, focusing awareness, optimism

Dharmachakra Mudra is a beautiful, outward expression of your innate desire to be loved for who you are. Practicing this mudra can teach you how to find harmony between your inner and outer worlds. As Brené Brown writes in *The Gifts of Imperfection*, "Authenticity is the daily practice of letting go of who we think we are supposed to be and embracing who we actually are." When your words, actions, and thoughts are aligned, you are living with integrity and authenticity.

When you love and accept your imperfections and quirks, you set an example of authentic self-love. You set down your masks and show up as your raw, imperfect self. And when you choose authenticity, you choose discomfort over discontentment. You say what is in your heart with honesty and integrity instead of holding on to discontentment and resentment.

Sometimes there is a large gap between who we are at our core and how we show up in the world. Somewhere along the way we lose sight of who we are and what makes our heart sing. Practice Dharmachakra Mudra if you feel like you've lost your way or you've lost touch with your essence, your true nature.

1. Dharmachakra Mudra is a beautiful mudra practiced with both hands. Bring your hands in front of your heart and turn your left palm toward your heart and your right palm away from it.
2. Bring the thumb and index finger of each hand to touch. Then, bring the tip of your left middle finger to where the right index finger and thumb meet.
3. A second version of Dharmachakra Mudra is often depicted in Buddhist iconography. This version brings the touching index finger and thumb of each hand to touch the tips of the opposite hand's index finger and thumb.
4. Hold for 10 to 30 minutes.

## Inner Self-Meditation

1. In a comfortable posture, either seated or lying down, take a moment to experience your breath in your belly. Notice its ebbs and flows. Notice where it flows freely and where it meets resistance.
2. Now bring your hands into Dharmachakra Mudra.

3. With each cycle of breath, envision dancing particles of light pouring into your crown chakra and down through your body into your core. This light fills you with peace, balance, and harmony.
4. Notice the muscles of your face, neck, and shoulders soften. Your masks fall away one piece at a time as your body fills with the radiant light of self-love, self-acceptance, and authenticity.
5. At your core, your center, you see who you are. Explore this inner self. Ask questions and allow them to be answered.
6. Stay with this meditation for 5 to 15 minutes.

## SPIRITUAL AWAKENING
### Garuda Mudra / Mythical Bird Gesture

**Chakras:** Crown, Heart, Solar Plexus, Third Eye, Throat

**Also good for:** commitment, increasing prana and vitality, intuition, perseverance, protection, relieving exhaustion and fatigue

Garuda, king of birds, master of air, devourer of snakes and poisons, shares his gifts in the form of safety, security, and self-acceptance. He awakens our ability to see the big picture and the minute details clearly. Garuda helps us see what's ahead so we can plan accordingly and he helps us trust our inner guide as we soar through this journey of life. Garuda offers strength and protection from poison and helps us cultivate our spirituality. We can ask Garuda for guidance when we're feeling lost and he will show us the way. Garuda Mudra can help us overcome self-doubt, self-criticism, and fear.

Garuda Mudra helps us on our path of spiritual awakening by increasing our ability to communicate with our spirit guides, and it opens us to receive their guidance. Practicing Garuda Mudra can help us see the path ahead clearly. This path of awakening leads us to a state of enlightenment characterized by inner peace, personal worth, unconditional happiness, and freedom from stress, worry, and anxiety.

1. Garuda Mudra can be practiced any time. Bring your hands in front of your heart. Turn the palms of your hands in toward your chest, cross your wrists, and interlace your thumbs.
2. Extend your remaining fingers out long and spread them wide.
3. Hold this mudra for 10 to 20 minutes.

## Eagle Meditation

1. Bring your hands into Garuda Mudra in front of your pelvis, navel, or heart. If your arms become tired, rest your hands on your heart.
2. Breathe deeply. Notice the rise and fall of your chest. Witness your breath as the vehicle of prana. Become aware of the flow of prana in your arms and hands.
3. Now envision a magnificent grove of trees. Within the trees you see a perfectly formed eagle's nest. You see three eagles soaring above you. You feel their presence as teachers and guides.
4. They invite you to join them on their flight. You, too, can soar. As you rise above the sacred Earth, feel the wind beneath your wings. Feel the warmth of the sun on your skin and the gentle breeze.
5. From this vantage point, the eagles show you your path. Travel along this path and follow its course. See the path as it meanders through forests, along cliffs, and over mountains. As you follow its course, you gain

Continued

insights and clarity. On this flight you realize you have unlimited access
to spirit.

6. Gently fly back to the grove of trees. Come back into your body. Feel
the weight of your bones, the fluctuations of your breath, and the sacred
rhythm of your heart.

7. Allow wisdom and insight to settle in.

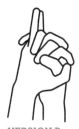

VERSION A     VERSION B

## TRANSFORMATION
### Kali Mudra / Goddess of Destruction Gesture

**Chakras:** Heart, Root, Solar Plexus, Third Eye, Throat

**Also good for:** clearing attachments and negativity, overcoming fear, purification, releasing limiting beliefs

Kali, the dark goddess of destruction and slayer of demons, is depicted with deep blue skin, wild hair, sharp teeth, and blood dripping from her long tongue. She wears a garland of skulls around her neck and a skirt made of bones. She is wild, fierce, and terrifying. She also loves unconditionally. She will fight our battles, slay our demons, and remove evil, ignorance, and ego from our lives, but she expects us to do the work, too. Goddess Kali and Kali Mudra give us the gift of transformation.

Kali Mudra teaches us about personal power, overcoming obstacles, protecting ourselves and loved ones, and loving unconditionally. We can call in the fierce goddess energy of Kali by practicing Kali Mudra when dealing with a particularly unbearable coworker, when needing to cultivate our fierce mother energy to protect our children, or when we face the same challenges repeatedly. When the energy of Kali is working in our lives, we actively release what no longer serves us: the emotional baggage, toxic relationships, and self-limiting beliefs that drag us down and keep us small. Practice Kali Mudra when you're ready for transformation.

There are two popular versions of Kali Mudra: With the index fingers extended long, it is used for matters of the heart and ego. With the ring fingers extended long, it addresses matters of the first chakra—overcoming first chakra fears; for example, feelings of lack, of not being safe.

### FOR VERSION A, TO ADDRESS MATTERS OF THE HEART AND EGO:

1. Bring the palms of your hands to touch in front of your heart. Interlace your fingers with your left thumb on top and extend your index fingers straight—imagine the extended index fingers as Kali's sword.
2. Practice this mudra for up to 45 minutes.

### FOR VERSION B, TO OVERCOME FIRST CHAKRA FEARS:

1. Bring the hands, again as in version A, in front of the heart. Keep your ring fingers extended while you interlace your remaining fingers, with your left thumb crossing over your right thumb.
2. Practice this mudra for up to 45 minutes.

## Kali Meditation

1. For this meditation practice, we'll channel the fierce goddess energy of Mother Kali.
2. Find a comfortable seated posture under the watchful guidance, unconditional love, and fierce protection of Kali; sit upright, strong, and confident.
3. Experience your breath in the back of your throat as you breathe in and out.
4. Now bring your hands into Kali Mudra at your heart center, or extend your arms overhead.
5. Chant "Om Krim Kalikayai Namaha" (pronounced *ohm kreem kah-lee-ka-yay nah-mah-hah*) 9, 27, 54, or 108 times (108 is a sacred number in yoga and Ayurveda, and 108 is divisible by 9, 27, and 54).
6. Bring your awareness back to your breath for a moment.
7. End with a few rounds of Lion's Breath, a fierce pranayama that increases prana, clears blockages, and cultivates the fierce energy of a lioness protecting her young. To practice Lion's Breath, breathe in through your nose and exhale forcefully through your mouth, stick out your tongue, and bug out your eyes. You might feel a little silly at first, but stay with it. Practice three to nine rounds.
8. Invite your mouth and eyes to close and take a minute or two to notice how you feel.

## HEART WISDOM
### Anjali Mudra / Divine Offering Gesture

**Chakras:** Crown, Heart

**Also good for:** balance, focus, respectful relationships, stress reduction, uniting body and mind

Anjali Mudra is an ancient Indian hand gesture and it may be the most widely used hand mudra today. Not only is it a salutation, it is also a sign of respect and an acknowledgement of the Divine within.

Anjali Mudra brings us back to the heart, so we may see the Divine within us all. This mudra helps us experience the interconnectedness of all beings. In Mark Nepo's *The Book of Awakening*, he shares the meaning of "Ubuntu," a South African saying that means "I am because you are; you are because I am." Ubuntu refers to our shared humanity characterized by kindness, compassion, and virtue. It recognizes the Divine and the humane within all of us, much like "namaste," which is a Sanskrit salutation, a sign of respect, and an opportunity to honor and recognize the Divine in another being.

Anjali Mudra moves us out of the thinking, analyzing mind and into the wisdom of the heart. You'll find Anjali Mudra helpful in matters of the heart, connection, and relationships. If you're experiencing a sense of separation or a lack of connection, practice Anjali Mudra to find unity and harmony.

I like to combine Anjali Mudra with namaste when I find myself struggling to see the Divine within others, like when getting cut off in traffic or dealing with challenging people. A quick Anjali + namaste is enough to remind me we're all doing the best we can with our current state of awareness. Anjali Mudra can be practiced anytime.

1. Bring your hands into "prayer position" in front of the heart, with the palms of your hands touching and fingers pointing up toward the heavens.
2. Practice Anjali Mudra as needed, for up to 45 minutes.

## Heart Wisdom Meditation

1. Take a seat, making sure your spine is long and your heart space is open—roll your shoulders back and down to broaden across your collarbones.
2. Bring your hands into Anjali Mudra. If you're seeking guidance in a specific relationship, endeavor, or life in general, take a moment to ask your heart for guidance.
3. Move your awareness to your breath in your heart space. Experience both your breath and your heart.

Continued

4. The air in your lungs and your breath unite as one. Sense this unity in the interconnectedness of all beings.

5. Now bring your awareness back to your heart. Your physical heart and your heartbeat.

6. Continue to follow your breath and your heart until you sense the connection with all beings. Listen closely to the wisdom of your heart. What is it telling you?

7. Experience fully the divinity in all beings.

8. Breathe slowly. Your being and all beings are filled with kindness, compassion, and virtue.

CHAPTER FOUR

# Live and Love

In our final chapter, you'll find mudras and meditations for bringing balance and healing to matters of the heart. This chapter focuses on self-care—and I'm not talking about hot baths and spa days (although those are great, too!). The ultimate self-care is practicing self-love, unconditional love. You'll find mudras to heal a broken heart, to trust your intuition, to accept what you cannot change, and change what you can. These mudras and meditations will ask you to expand, to get a little uncomfortable, to clear out the toxic parts of your life to make space for your truth, for courageous love, and creative self-expression.

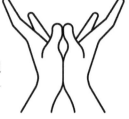

## SELF-LOVE
### Padma Mudra / Lotus Seal

**Chakras:** Heart, Root, Sacral

**Also good for:** affection and compassion, faith, living your truth, personal growth, resilience, wisdom

Padma Mudra is known as the lotus mudra, or lotus seal, and it is a beautiful mudra to incorporate into a meditation or asana practice. In Sanskrit, *padma* is commonly translated as "lotus" or "sacred lotus." Lotus Mudra teaches us to lean into the strength of our roots, to have faith in the journey, to be loving and kind on the path. The sacred lotus helps us see the beauty of our soul and reminds us of the Divine within.

Lotus symbolism and imagery is common throughout Hinduism, Sikhism, Jainism, and Buddhism. A lotus flower takes root down in the muck and mud and rises up through the water to blossom, beautiful and unscathed, at the water's surface. Like the lotus, our journey toward enlightenment grows from the darkness of fear and ignorance to blossom in the light of love and self-realization.

Practice Padma Mudra when you need help believing in your potential, when you feel emotionally drained, or when you need to remember that you, too, are worthy of love.

1. Practice Padma Mudra by bringing your hands in front of your heart with your palms touching in "prayer position." Keep the heels of your hands, thumbs, and pinky fingers touching and pull your index, middle, and ring fingers and palms away from one another.
2. Hold this mudra for 15 to 45 minutes.

## Self-Love Meditation

1. Find a comfortable seated posture. If you have healthy knees and open hips, you could even try sitting in half lotus or full lotus, although any seated posture will do. Your first act of self-love is to make sure the posture you choose is nourishing and easeful.
2. Bring your hands into Padma Mudra in front of your heart. Close your eyes and steady your breath. Take a moment simply to breathe. Hear the hum of your breath as you breathe in and out.
3. Now bring your awareness to your heart space and see a beautiful pink lotus blossom at the center of your chest. This lotus flower is symbolic of your awakening heart chakra. Envision the petals opening to receive Divine love. The blossom of the lotus resembles a chalice. Each inhale breath fills the chalice of the open lotus with love, compassion, affection,

Continued

faith, and joy. Each exhale flows down your spine, down the stem of the lotus, into its roots to nourish others. There is a constant stream of love.

4. Now choose one of the following affirmations or create your own to repeat:

I am worthy of love. I am love.

I am resilient. I am capable.

My heart is wide open. I am worthy of love, compassion, joy, and affection.

## UNSHAKEABLE TRUST

Vajrapradama Mudra /
Unshakeable Trust Gesture

**Chakras:** Heart

**Also good for:** commitment, communicating with love and courage, faith in and connection to something greater, navigating life transitions, opening the heart, self-confidence, self-love, self-truth

Vajrapradama Mudra is a powerful mudra to help you transcend feelings of self-doubt, unworthiness, self-loathing, and fear in its various forms.

I like to practice Vajrapradama in meditation, in yoga poses, and even before having difficult conversations with loved ones and coworkers. This mudra helps you tap right into the heart for compassionate communication, trust in yourself, and faith that your words will be delivered gracefully and received openly.

This mudra teaches us to trust. In particular, it teaches us to trust our self. When we trust our self, we show up in the world with a calm, gentle confidence. We are courageous. Do you know where the word *courage* comes from? Author Brené Brown explains courage as "a heart word. The root of the word courage is *cor*, the Latin word for *heart*. In one of its earliest forms, the word courage meant 'to speak one's mind by telling all one's heart.'" The root of the word courage rests in our ability to trust the wisdom of our heart, to trust it's okay to show up vulnerably, and to trust that our vulnerability will be met with respect.

1. Bring your hands in front of your heart and interlace your fingers. Separate your palms and place your open hands over your heart space. Your thumbs will point upward.
2. This mudra can be practiced in any posture for as long as necessary.

## Heart Meditation

1. For this meditation, you will be in a supported heart-opener position. You will need a blanket or thick towel. Roll the blanket into a roll two to three feet long. Place this rolled blanket on the floor or on a yoga mat behind you. Take a seat at the skinny end of your blanket roll and then lie on the blanket roll so it is aligned with your spine. If your head is not supported, tuck another blanket or pillow underneath your head. Invite your shoulders to soften down toward the floor. This posture creates space in the front of the chest, improves posture, and helps open the heart.
2. Bring your hands into Vajrapradama Mudra. Close your eyes and breathe into your heart space. Feel the rise and fall of your breath beneath your hands. Witness your breath and invite it to deepen. Trust that each exhale will be followed by an inhale.

3. Stay with your breath. If any thoughts bubble up to the surface, take a moment to explore them without judgment, attachment, or expectation.
4. Trust your inner wisdom, the wisdom of your heart. You are more knowledgeable than you give yourself credit for. Allow inner wisdom to wash over you.
5. Stay with this meditation for 5 to 10 minutes.

## ACCEPTANCE
**Pushpaputa Mudra /
Handful of Flowers Gesture**

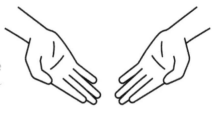

**Chakras:** Heart, Root, Sacral

**Also good for:** compassion, emotional balance, gratitude, overcoming fear, promoting positivity and optimism, receptivity, spacious heart and mind

What does it mean to practice acceptance? Eckhart Tolle, author of *A New Earth*, explains acceptance as when "you allow yourself to feel whatever it is you are feeling at that moment. It is part of the *isness* of the Now. You can't argue with what is. Well, you can, but if you do, you suffer."

Acceptance is an active practice that takes continual effort. Acceptance is not apathy. Nor does practicing acceptance mean you're endorsing that which is out of your control. Nor does it mean you cannot change.

You've likely heard the popular saying from Carl Jung, "What we resist persists." When we constantly battle that which is out of our control, we suffer; the quality of our mind is disturbed. What we can control are our actions and responses. Remember, acceptance is a practice and, for most of us, it takes consistent effort to achieve results. When you show up in the world and practice acceptance and compassion, you are a beacon of light for others.

In Pushpaputa Mudra, the hands resemble an empty bowl symbolizing our receptivity to knowledge and wisdom. *Pushpaputa*, in Sanskrit, means "handful of flowers," which represents an offering to a higher power. There is a balance between giving and receiving. What we give is what we receive. This mudra awakens us to the flow of energy, the give and take that occurs at all times, the microcosm within the macrocosm.

Practice Pushpaputa Mudra daily as a reminder to practice acceptance, or practice it when things aren't working out as you want—when life throws you curveballs. This mudra can help you find calm, peace, and contentment, and help you see you have all you need within you and around you. Acceptance is practicing radical self-love as you learn to love your darkness, your shadow, and everything you cannot change.

1. Place your hands in your lap and turn the palms of your hands facing upward. The hands are gently open with the fingers and thumbs close to one another.
2. Practice Pushpaputa Mudra for up to 45 minutes per day.

## Seeking versus Seeing Meditation

1. For this meditation, go outside and find a comfortable seat or a spot where you can recline on the Earth. Your eyes will remain open for the majority of this meditation.

Continued

2. Bring your hands into Pushpaputa Mudra and peer up at the sky. Watch the clouds and find a cloud that looks like a rabbit.

3. Continue watching the clouds and now choose a cloud to witness. What shapes arise?

4. Close your eyes and take a moment to reflect on the difference between seeking something and seeing what is there.

## LETTING GO
Ksepana Mudra / Gesture to Let Go

**Chakras:** Heart, Root, Sacral

**Also good for:** purification, surrendering to the flow of life, release from suffering, negativity, and tension

We spend many precious hours holding on to the things we like and avoiding things we don't. We attach to loved ones—and when they leave us, we suffer. We attach to our favorite meal at our favorite restaurant—and when they change the menu, we suffer. When our aversion to spiders causes us to smash an unsuspecting spider, we cause suffering. Ksepana Mudra is about the practice of letting go and releasing the attachments of the ego.

You may also find practicing Ksepana Mudra can help you navigate a changing relationship or stressful situation. If I'm super stressed, Ksepana Mudra can help me release my perfectionist tendencies and be a little kinder and gentler with myself. Now when I practice Ksepana Mudra I instantly enter a calmer, clearer state of being.

Ksepana Mudra should be practiced when you're ready to be free of attachments and negativity. With continued practice, you'll likely start decluttering and letting go of the physical and emotional baggage in your life and emerge with a weight lifted off your shoulders. Practice Ksepana

Mudra when you're ready to step into the joy, bliss, and contentment of an awakened life.

1. To practice Ksepana Mudra, bring the palms of your hands together to touch. Interlace your fingers, cross your thumbs, and, finally, extend your index fingers long. Turn the index fingers to point down toward the ground or your feet.
2. Hold for as long as desired.

## Waterfall Meditation

1. Find a comfortable seated position in which you are able to sit tall with your rib cage stacked effortlessly over your hips.
2. Bring your hands into Ksepana Mudra and allow your hands and arms to rest gently in your lap, with your index fingers pointing down toward the ground.
3. Close your eyes and take a few deep, cleansing breaths—in through your nose and out through your mouth.
4. Inhale and mindfully sweep your arms forward and up toward the sky and imagine gathering warm, vibrant, healing energy.
5. When you exhale, the warm vibrant energy you have gathered pours over your body like a gently flowing waterfall. As you exhale, allow your thumbs to gently trace a line from the crown of your head to the bridge

of your nose, across your chin, down through your heart center, and back to your pelvis. With each exhale breath you let go of negativity, fear, emotional baggage, and attachments. The gentle water of the falls clears away the debris of habits, thoughts, and toxic relationships that no longer serve you.

6. Continue to connect your breath with the movement of the mudra and the visualization.

7. Repeat as many rounds as necessary. When you feel complete, return to the starting position and take a few moments to sit in stillness. Take this time to notice the effects of your meditation practice.

## HEART-CENTERED RELATIONSHIPS
Anahata Chakra Mudra /
Heart Chakra Gesture

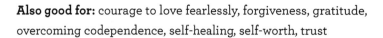

**Chakras:** Heart

**Also good for:** courage to love fearlessly, forgiveness, gratitude, overcoming codependence, self-healing, self-worth, trust

The Anahata Chakra Mudra awakens our heart chakra. When our heart chakra is open and balanced, we find it easy to be loving and compassionate and our relationships are healthy and heart-centered. If you're in a season of life that feels emotionally out of balance (e.g., you're reactive, quick to anger, jealous, or resentful), practicing Anahata Chakra Mudra can help blossom the lotus of your heart chakra and guide you back to a place of self-love, grace, and acceptance.

Anahata Chakra Mudra can also be helpful if you're feeling lonely, isolated, disconnected from your loved ones, or you're healing a broken heart. Just a few moments each morning can set the tone for the rest of your day. You'll notice your communication is rooted in love, you vibrate at a higher frequency, you attract those who are vibrating at the same level, and you'll find it easier to practice love, gratitude, and acceptance.

It's easy to recognize the people in your life whose heart chakra is open because they radiate love in all they do. Love emanates from their eyes.

They're unfazed by life's challenges. They're genuine and altruistic and they love others unconditionally.

1. Anahata Chakra Mudra is practiced by bringing the hands in front of your heart with the tips of your fingers touching.
2. Bring the tips of your ring fingers into the webbing between the middle and index fingers of the opposite hand and then curl your middle fingers over your ring fingers. You'll see a heart shape.
3. Hold this mudra for 20 minutes, or for as long is comfortable.

## Gratitude Meditation

I encourage you to create a daily gratitude practice. Daily gratitude helps us cultivate love and appreciation for others and ourselves. Practice this gratitude meditation each morning or evening.

1. Bring your hands into Anahata Chakra Mudra in front of your heart.
2. Take a few rounds of expansive breath. Allow this breath to drop you into your heart and, as you drop into your heart, drop into your physical body. Experience the weight of your bones, the expansion and contraction of your ribs. Invite a sense of stillness and peace to wash into your body.

Continued

3. As you sit here, feel every cell vibrate with contentment, love, and peace as you begin your gratitude practice.

4. What are you grateful for? Today I am grateful for _____.

5. Keep repeating, "Today I am grateful for _____." Take a moment of gratitude for the tiny, mundane things in your life as well as the large, complex things. Find gratitude for the parts of your life that are easy to be grateful for, and for the parts of your life that are a challenge to be grateful for. And be grateful for everything in between.

6. Eventually, shorten the statement to "I am grateful."

7. And then, "I am gratitude."

# HEALTHY WRISTS AND SHOULDERS

1. In a comfortable seated position, bring your hands to your knees. On an inhale breath, tilt your pelvis forward, arch your back, lift your chest up toward the sky, and turn your gaze upward. On an exhale, tuck your chin toward your chest, round your spine, and tuck your tailbone under. Stretch the space between your shoulder blades. Take 5 to 10 rounds to release tension in your shoulders and back.
2. Sit tall and stretch your right fingertips out and down toward the floor. Then draw your left ear toward your left shoulder. Breathe here for three to five rounds of breath; repeat on the other side.
3. Interlace your hands behind your back with the palms of your hands touching and lift your chest.
4. Interlace your hands in front of you and extend your arms long. Turn your palms to face away from you and, alternately, raise and lower your left and right wrists an inch or two. Retain the bind and stretch your arms up overhead. Breathe here for a moment. Release your arms out and down to the sides and make circles with your wrists as you lower them.
5. Finally, give each of your forearms, wrists, and hands a quick massage.

## FEARLESS LOVE
Abhaya Hridaya Mudra /
Fearless Heart Gesture

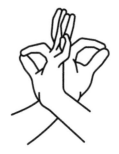

**Chakras:** Heart, Solar Plexus

**Also good for:** calming strong emotions, connecting to your truth, emotional healing, overcoming resistance and self-doubt, reassurance and safety, releasing stress

Love transcends all. Love is where we came from and love is where we'll return. Whether your heart has been broken by a recent breakup or you're holding on to an old fear from childhood, this mudra can help you find the space in your heart to love again and heal from past pains and traumas. This mudra brings you back home to your essence, your truth, and the abundance of love.

*Abhaya* means "without fear" in Sanskrit. This mudra encourages us to follow our heart, even if it might get messy and uncomfortable. When we're cruising in our comfort zone, we're living a life guided by fear.

We fear being seen, making mistakes, and getting hurt. Abhaya Hridaya Mudra will help you crack open the hard, protective shell of your heart to let the light in—the light of love, compassion, trust, and freedom. Fear keeps us small and contracted. Fear sabotages our relationships and steals from our futures.

I was recently reflecting on how fear robs us of love. A friend waited to come out to his dad until he was 30. Fear had prevented him from sharing himself fully with his father. When he came out, his father still loved him and they're now closer than ever. Loving fearlessly means loving through uncertainty and discomfort.

1. Bring the backs of your hands to touch like a "reverse prayer position" and interlace your middle, ring, and pinky fingers.
2. Then bring the tips of your index fingers to touch the tips of your thumbs.
3. Hold for 5 to 15 minutes.

## Fearless Love Meditation

1. Find an upright, comfortable seat. Close your eyes and bring your hands into Abhaya Hridaya Mudra.
2. Imagine someone who radiates love, who loves you unconditionally, sitting right in front of you. This person could be a parent, friend, child, pet, teacher, or guru.

Continued

3. Now imagine a bright white light flowing from their heart to your heart. This radiant light fills your heart with unconditional love. Your heart is filled with love that knows no bounds. Release any resistance to receiving this love. You are worthy of love. Feel a weight lifted off your shoulders. Feel tension release from your face. Feel your heart soften.

4. Experience this lightness, your heart bathed in radiant love.

5. From this place of abundant love, it is your turn to share love. See someone in front of you who needs love. This person could be someone you love, someone who challenges you, or it could be a group of people.

6. Send loving white light straight from your heart into theirs. See a weight lifted off their shoulders. See tension release from their face. See them soften into love.

## SELF-EXPRESSION AND CREATIVITY
### Udana Vayu Mudra /
### Upward Moving Air Gesture

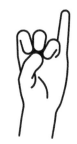

**Chakras:** Heart, Root, Solar Plexus, Throat

**Also good for:** confidence, focus, joy, optimism, prosperity, spiritual growth, taste and smell, wisdom

Udana Vayu Mudra helps us honor and hone our creative expression. This mudra helps regulate the flow of Udana Vayu, which is the upward flow of energy in the chest, throat, and head. It also helps activate the throat chakra, our center of creative expression, communication, and the outward expression of our individuality.

An imbalance in Udana Vayu can cause issues with voice and speech, self-expression, shortness of breath, depression, and even memory retention and mental sharpness.

Self-expression is available to us once we have done the work of the third and fourth chakras, when we're confident in our self-worth and we practice unconditional self-love. The next time you have a creative project, whether it's a work project, painting, writing, making something, or cooking from scratch, take a moment beforehand to practice Udana Vayu Mudra and you'll tap into your creative potential.

If expressing yourself seems daunting, know that many people seek your gifts. By playing small and safe, you withhold your talents from the world; some would say you're being selfish! Get out there, share your creativity, share your dharma, share your joy, and watch it light up the community around you.

Practice something each day that brings you joy, that elevates your vibration. Don't be afraid to create, to make mistakes, to speak your truth, or to live big. This one and only life you are living is your canvas and you are the masterpiece, so make it glorious.

1. To practice Udana Vayu Mudra, bring the tips of your index, middle, and ring fingers to touch the tips of your thumbs. Extend your pinky fingers long.
2. This mudra can be practiced anytime for 15 to 30 minutes at a time.

## Udana Vayu Meditation

We'll begin this meditation practice with an audible humming pranayama called Brahmari. Brahmari is also known as bumblebee breath because the sound of the exhale sounds just like the buzz of a bumblebee.

1. Find a comfortable seated position, close your eyes, and take a few centering breaths.

2. Breathe in through your nose. On your exhale, breathe out through your nose while humming and rocking your jaw side to side. Repeat 5 to 10 times.

3. Notice the subtle vibration in your skull. You may even notice a shift in energy in your head and throat. You feel positive and light.

4. Now bring your awareness to your throat and your fifth chakra, Vishuddha. Envision a vibrant turquoise-blue lotus flower. Hold this visualization.

5. Now meditate on the throat as the sound of the cosmos and the center of your creative expression. Continue to hold your awareness at your throat chakra for the duration of the meditation.

6. Practice for 5 to 10 minutes.

## EXPANSION / PERSONAL GROWTH
### Vyana Mudra /
### Outward Flowing Gesture

**Chakras:** Heart, Throat

**Also good for:** assertiveness and enthusiasm, comfort and healing, connection with others, coordination, elimination of toxins via sweat and bowel movements, improving balance, locomotion, love, mental stability

Vyana Mudra is all about expansion. Vyana Mudra regulates the flow of Vyana Vayu, the air or energy in the body that flows from the center out into the extremities. By practicing Vyana Mudra, we embody the expansive qualities of Vyana Vayu.

Practicing Vyana Mudra can bring harmony to the path of expansion. When we're in a period of expansion, it can be uncomfortable. Actually, if I'm honest, expanding oneself can be incredibly uncomfortable and it may even make you want to run for the hills! When you're expanding yourself, you're constantly pushing up against your edges, working through those edges, and creating new edges. Vyana Mudra can help you stay mentally alert and agile as you learn new skills, or new ways of being.

When we start something new, whether it's a new project or a new relationship, it's exciting and fresh and we feel enthusiastic. However, as time goes on, we sometimes end up burned-out, exhausted, and bored.

The next time you feel like you've fallen out of love (with a person or a project), practice Vyana Mudra to bring back enthusiasm and excitement. During this phase of expansion, anxiety might creep in and your sleep might suffer. If you experience anxiety, I recommend practicing Vyana Mudra first thing in the morning and when you crawl into bed at night.

1. With each hand, bring the tip of your index and middle fingers to meet the tip of your thumb. Extend your ring and pinky fingers out long.
2. Practice Vyana Mudra for 5 to 50 minutes.

## Vyana Vayu Meditation

1. For this meditation, you can sit, lie down, or stand. Bring your hands into Vyana Mudra and rest the backs of your hands on your thighs. Close your eyes. Breathe slowly and deeply for a few minutes.
2. Keep your hands in Vyana Mudra and bring them in front of your chest.
3. On your inhale breath, extend your arms out to the side. Retain your breath and feel energy, prana, flowing from your heart out through your arms, crown, hips, legs, and beyond.
4. As you exhale, bring your hands back in front of your chest and feel the energy return to your heart center.

Continued

5. Witness this sacred expansion and contraction, called *spanda*, which is often translated as the pulse, vibration, or throb originating simultaneously from our center and from everywhere at once.
6. Practice 10 to 15 rounds of breath and then return the backs of your hands to your thighs.
7. Take a few more moments to witness the natural flow of energy.
8. When you're ready, allow your eyes to flutter open softly.

## PERSONAL TRUTH

Avahana Mudra / Summoning Gesture

**Chakras:** Heart, Solar Plexus

**Also good for:** acceptance, forgiveness, inner guidance, invoking the Divine/deity, mental brightness

*Avahana* means "to summon" in Sanskrit. Avahana Mudra is used to invoke a deity in devotional practice. It is also used to call forth our inner truth. This mudra can be helpful when navigating challenging situations, managing "energy vampires," and clearing away distractions. With Avahana Mudra, we can sit in the light of our inner truth. Avahana Mudra helps us find a state of *svastha*, or well-being. When our body is well, our mind is clear, and we're free from outside distractions and attachments, it's easier to access the limitlessness of our true nature, of the Divine light within.

When you're steady in your inner truth, life's curve balls won't rattle you as badly and you'll recover more quickly. It's easier for us to come back to our center because it's familiar. Being steady in your inner truth requires self-love, self-acceptance, and forgiveness. When you're unshakeable in your inner truth, it's easier to see the Divine in all things and all situations. It's easier to see the blessings and gifts each moment provides, blessings in the ease and joy as well as the blessings in the moments of growth.

Practice Avahana Mudra when you feel like you've given up so much of yourself to fit in or be loved that you've lost your center and inner light. Practice Avahana Mudra to fill up your "love cup" and embrace your authentic self and inner truth.

1. Place your upward-facing palms in your lap and, on each hand, bring the tip of your thumb to the base of your pinky finger. All other fingers are extended softly.
2. Hold for 15 to 30 minutes.

## Inner Flame Meditation

1. Practice Avahana Mudra in a comfortable seat, either propped up on a cushion or sitting with your feet firmly planted on the ground.
2. Bring your hands into Avahana Mudra with the pinky-sides of your hands touching. Here you can either let your hands rest in your lap or hold them in front of your navel.
3. Close your eyes and fold the palms of your hands toward one another. Begin to deepen your breath. Practice five to seven rounds of Square Breath (page 16).
4. Keep your hands in Avahana Mudra with the palms folded in toward one another and bring your hands in front of your heart. The hands will

resemble a candle flame. This flame represents the light of your inner truth. It burns continuously.

5. Envision the flame of your inner truth glowing brightly. Each cycle of breath fans the flames and the flame grows even brighter.
6. Hold your awareness here and explore the depths of your inner light, of your truth, of your center.
7. Hold the vision of the flame in your mind's eye for another 5 to 10 minutes.
8. Afterward, release the mudra and give yourself another moment to sit quietly.

# UNION OF OPPOSITES
## Makara Mudra / Crocodile Gesture

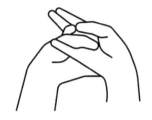

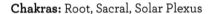

**Chakras:** Root, Sacral, Solar Plexus

**Also good for:** calm, concentration, forgiveness, improving memory, relieving tension and lower back pain, restoring vitality, stress relief

The Makara is a mythical Indian crocodile who carries the goddess Ganga. The crocodile is both fierce and still, hard and soft, explosive and tender, and capable on land and water. The crocodile is rough, jagged, and sharp at its surface, but its underbelly is soft and tender. Aren't we the same at times? Makara Mudra channels and unites these opposing energies and teaches us we can balance action and stillness, strength and softness.

Practicing Makara Mudra restores our energy reserves and helps us access our hidden potential that lies beneath the surface. Practice Makara Mudra the next time your energy reserves feel low, whether you're a parent acting as chauffeur/chef/nurse/superhero, a university student in the middle of finals week, or it's the darkest days of winter and you just need a little boost. Makara Mudra can also be helpful when you feel dissatisfied with life or are holding on to an old grudge. It can help clear out old emotions stored in your first and second chakras.

1. Makara Mudra is practiced with both hands. With your right hand, curl your right ring finger in and place your right thumb pad over the top of the ring finger fingernail.
2. With your left hand, bring your left thumb to the palm of your right hand and wrap the fingers of your left hand around the back of your right hand.
3. Hold for up to 30 minutes.

## A Balance of Opposites Meditation

1. Come into a comfortable seated position. For this meditation, we begin with a pranayama called *nadi shodhana*, or alternate nostril breathing. Nadi shodhana helps balance the right and left hemispheres of the brain and helps clear the energy channels known as nadis.
2. With your right hand, bring your thumb to your right nostril, your ring finger to your left nostril, and place your index finger and middle finger gently on your third eye.
3. Close your eyes. Take a full breath in. Then exhale and block your right nostril while breathing out through your left nostril. Inhale through your left nostril. Block your left nostril and exhale through the right nostril.

Continued

Inhale through your right nostril. That is one full round. To simplify, inhale, then:

**Block right; exhale left**
**Inhale left**
**Block left; exhale right**
**Inhale right**

4. Complete 10 to 15 rounds of nadi shodhana.
5. With your eyes still closed, bring your hands into Makara Mudra.
6. With each inhale breath, imagine your breath, the vehicle of prana, as a steady stream of light flowing in through your nostrils and to your third eye. Hold awareness at your third eye as you breathe out.
7. In your mind's eye, imagine yourself as a Makara, a crocodile. Experience both the softness of your underbelly and the fierceness of your potential.

# Resources

*The Book of Awakening: Having the Life You Want by Being Present to the Life You Have* **by Mark Nepo**

*Guided Meditations, Explorations, and Healings* **by Stephen Levine**

*Hatha Yoga Pradipika* **by Swami Muktibodhananda**

*Healing Mantras* **by Thomas Ashley-Farrand**

*Mudras for Modern Life: Boost Your Health, Re-Energize Your Life, Enhance Your Yoga, and Deepen Your Meditation* **by Swami Saradananda**

*Mudras of Yoga: 72 Hand Gestures for Healing and Spiritual Growth* **by Cain Carroll with Revital Carroll**

*Mudras: Yoga in Your Hands* **by Gertrud Hirschi**

# References

**Bradford, Alina.** "Lungs: Facts, Function, and Diseases." *Live Science*. February 2, 2018. www.livescience.com/52250-lung.html.

**Brown, Brené.** *I Thought It Was Just Me: Women Reclaiming Power and Courage in a Culture of Shame*. New York: Penguin Publishing Group, 2007.

    —*The Gifts of Imperfection: Let Go of Who You Think You're Supposed to Be and Embrace Who You Are*. Center City, MN: Hazelden Publishing, 2010.

**Carroll, Cain.** *Mudras of Yoga: 72 Hand Gestures for Healing and Spiritual Growth*. Philadelphia: Singing Dragon, 2014.

**Church, Dawson.** "Tap Your Way to Healing with EFT." *Omega*. September 20, 2013. www.eomega.org/article/tap-your-way-to-healing-with-eft.

**Church, Dawson, et al.** "Psychological Trauma Symptom Improvement in Veterans Using EFT (Emotional Freedom Techniques): A Randomized Controlled Trial." *Journal of Nervous and Mental Disease* 201, no. 2 (2013): 153–160. doi.org/10.1097/NMD.0b013e31827f6351.

**Church, D., and J. Palmer-Hoffman.** "TBI Symptoms Improve after PTSD Remediation with Emotional Freedom Techniques." *Traumatology* 20, no. 3 (2014): 172–181. doi.org/10.1037/h0099831.

**Clarke, T., P. Barnes, L. Black, et al.** "Use of Yoga, Meditation, and Chiropractors Among U.S. Adults Aged 18 and Over." *National Center for Health Statistics Data Brief*, no. 325, Hyattsville, MD: NCHS, 2018. www.cdc.gov/nchs/data/databriefs/db325-h.pdf.

**Fields, Helen.** "The Gut: Where Bacteria and Immune System Meet." *Johns Hopkins Medicine*. November 2015. www.hopkinsmedicine.org/research/advancements-in-research/fundamentals/in-depth/the-gut-where-bacteria-and-immune-system-meet.

**Hanh, Thich Nhat.** *Peace Is Every Breath: A Practice for Our Busy Lives.* New York: HarperCollins, 2011.

**Hirschi, Gertrud.** *Mudras: Yoga in Your Hands.* Trans. Christine M. Grimm. York Beach, ME: Samuel Weiser, Inc., 2000.

**Johari, Harish.** *Chakras, Energy Centers of Transformation.* Rochester: Destiny Books, 2000.

**Lung Institute.** "Lung Capacity: What Does It Mean?" *Exhale* (blog). May 3, 2017. www.lunginstitute.com/blog/lung-capacity-what-does-it-mean.

**McGreevey, Sue.** "Eight Weeks to a Better Brain." *The Harvard Gazette.* January 21, 2011. https://news.harvard.edu/gazette/story/2011/01/eight -weeks-to-a-better-brain.

**Muktibodhananda, Swami.** *Hatha Yoga Pradipika.* Bihar, India: Yoga Publications Trust, 2013.

**Myss, Caroline.** *Anatomy of the Spirit: The Seven Stages of Power and Healing.* New York: Harmony Books, 1996.

**Nepo, Mark.** *The Book of Awakening: Having the Life You Want by Being Present to the Life You Have.* San Francisco: Conari Press, 2011.

**Saoji, Apar.** "Effects of Yogic Breath Regulation: A Narrative Review of Scientific Evidence." *Journal of Ayurveda and Integrative Medicine* 10, no. 1 (2019): 50–58. www.sciencedirect.com/science/article/pii /S0975947617303224.

**Saradananda, Swami.** *Mudras for Modern Life: Boost Your Health, Re-Energize Your Life, Enhance Your Yoga, and Deepen Your Meditation.* London: Watkins Media Limited, 2015.

**Shyam Karthik, P.** "Effect of Pranayama and Suryanamaskar on Pulmonary Functions in Medical Students." *Journal of Clinical and Diagnostic Research* 8, no. 12 (2014): BC04–BC06. doi.org/10.7860/ JCDR/2014/10281.5344.

**The Tapping Solution.** "What Is Tapping and How Can I Start Using It?" *The Tapping Solution.* Accessed September 23, 2019. www.thetappingsolution .com/what-is-eft-tapping.

**Tlalka, Stephany.** "Meditation Is the Fastest Growing Health Trend in America." *Mindful.* December 11, 2018. www.mindful.org/meditation -is-the-fastest-growing-health-trend-in-america.

**Tolle, Eckhart.** *A New Earth: Awakening to Your Life's Purpose.* New York: Penguin, 2005.

**Wu, Hsin-Jung.** "The Role of Gut Microbiota in Immune Homeostasis and Autoimmunity." *Gut Microbes* 3, no. 1 (2012): 4–14. doi.org/10.4161/ gmic.19320.

# Index

# About the Author

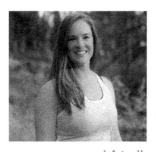

**Autumn Adams** is an international yoga teacher, based in Bend, Oregon. In 2014 her love of teaching yoga inspired her to create Ambuja Yoga, an online yoga resource for both yoga teachers and students. Through her teachings of yoga, shakti, mudras, and Ayurveda, she hopes to empower you to be courageous, to uncover your life's dharma, and to flow through life's challenges with grace and ease. She completed her 200-hour yoga teacher training with Jeannie Laslo Douglas in Bend, Oregon, and her 300-hour yoga teacher training with Zuna Yoga in Bali. Autumn also leads group yoga classes, nature-inspired transformational retreats, habit evolution courses, and yoga teacher trainings.